Around
the House

One Woman Shares
How Millions Care

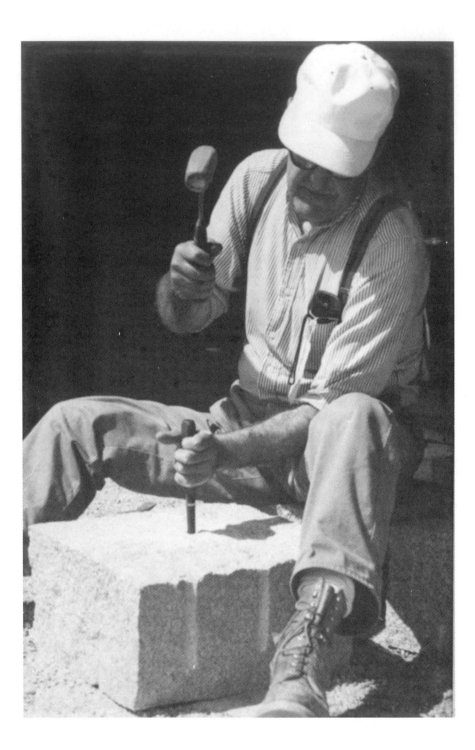

AROUND
the HOUSE

One Woman Shares
How Millions Care

By Harriet K. Swenson

Published by
Peter E. Randall Publisher
Portsmouth, New Hampshire
2015

ISBN 13: 978-1-942155-01-0
Library of Congress control number: 2014949085

Published by
Peter E. Randall Publisher
PO Box 4726
Portsmouth, NH 03802
www.perpublisher.com

Distributed by
University Press of New England
Lebanon, NH 03766
www.upne.com

Book design: Grace Peirce (nhmuse.com)

Frontispiece photo by Ray Snow, used with permission.

Contents

Definition of caregiver:
> Any person who cares for an individual needing help taking care of himself, in ways that range from meeting the basic needs of everyday life to offering medicine, nursing, or hospice care. Caregivers may be paid or volunteer; they include family and friends as well as doctors, nurses, social service providers, and hospice professionals.
> —from *Taking Care: Ethical Caregiving in Our Aging Society*, by The President's Council on Bioethics

Preface

My children tell me I worry too much. Perhaps I just keep things bottled up and only do a lot of stewing or speculating. But it is difficult to write about losing a loved one. It is especially difficult because I am a New Englander, and we are not known for talking out loud about so-called private or family matters. But when my beloved husband, David, received a serious diagnosis, I changed my tune. I took my years of frantic scribbled notes and turned them into short reflective unconventional responses to ordinary daily things. They do not contain depressing medical jargon and dreary academic facts. They are my silent, inner feelings of the moment.

The focus on the caregiver, not the patient, is the purpose here. The setting is picturesque New Hampshire. I mention places of escape, changed priorities, waivering faith, regional beaches, tender moments, Yankee frugality—the important things that a caregiver might not dare to talk about. But I gritted my teeth and did it, moving from romance to acute grief and the affirmation of what real love can do.

I. Beginnings

Partial to picnics in scenic places, my parents often drove us up to the Franconia Notch area of New Hampshire accompanied by a mammoth lunch of yummy deviled eggs, hearty meatloaf sandwiches, giant pickles, and my mother's famous crunchy molasses cookies all lovingly tucked into our worn wooden basket. They wanted us to gaze up at the Great Stone Face natural rock formation silhouetted against the bright blue sky. It was an image that had inspired all sorts of responses through the years, from Nathaniel Hawthorne's tale about a town trying to find a human match to the rugged face, to Daniel Webster's quip that the face was "a sign that in New Hampshire, God Almighty makes real men!"

Well, the rare landmark hadn't impressed me at all. As a child I had looked up and shuddered. Who cared? The lunch was great, but the stone face seemed remote, unexciting, overrated. When, in spite of diligent care and maintenance, the giant visage fell apart in May of 2003, friends actually called to say that the rocky formation had always reminded them of my husband, David. I was not surprised. He had died in February of the same year, and the rock's remembrance had at last fired up a powerful image for me.

David and I had been madly in love. A real New Englander, nonconformist and practical, he was good at repairing porch screens, and I had been good at making two children's dresses out of fabric intended for one. We were not as frugal, however, as the fellow who was rumored to have driven his car into his barn daily and jacked it up off the ground to save wear on the tires! But enough of that. I am on my way to a writers' workshop, which is a grand new experience to me, and I am feeling the usual rush of incompetency—call it what you will—in anticipation of all those "experts" who will of course be there. It is going to be given at one of my favorite places in the world, Star Island, part of the Isles of Shoals, nine miles off Portsmouth, New Hampshire, at the family vacation center. For many years our children and grandchildren and now great-grandchildren experience fresh air and the richness of healthy fellowship and fun, the quaint island harbor, the view from the old porch rocking chairs, the pitcher and bowl routine of washing up, the relaxed ambiance of a rare mix of people.

Yes, I'm old, too. Like the Great Stone Face. Maybe you noticed.

David and I met when I was fifty-one, he fifty-three. And yes, this is a love story; there wasn't a dry eye at our February wedding. But I'm getting ahead of my story.

We were under the illusion that New England frugality and modest expertise would make everything and everybody last forever, and love, sweat, and good intentions could ignore elements of chance, accident, mystery, evil, and misbehavior. Sickness in particular would never be part of our lives. It is only when a medical crisis hits that we plain ordinary people are jarred into paying attention to what has been creeping up on us, and once you've run up against modern health care issues, you and your family are never the same. When you are expected to understand the medical world with its high-tech advances, its abbreviated jargon, its obscene bills, and what my father called "those new fangled treatments," you find you run smack up against complex medical forms, coded print on midget pill bottles, and scary emergency room visits. In the 1950s at age twenty, I had known how to attract a tall Beta offering his frat pin come Saturday night, but more recently I had not figured out how to tackle the health care system. Even the word "medicine" had taken on puzzling meanings. Consider:

I gulped at the phrase "practice medicine." Does it mean they are using us as guinea pigs?

I winced at the phrase "boutique medicine." Does it include beads and trendy outerwear?

I woke up to the phrase "alternative medicine." It sounded better than needles.

Just yesterday I spotted reference to "narrative medicine." Do they talk you to death?

Of course, when two people find each other and they fall in love, they "make do," and we did. By the time I was "trying out" the Episcopal ten o'clock service at St. Paul's Church in Concord, New Hampshire, I had learned that the good-looking brown-haired fellow peering down at me over his tortoiseshell half-glasses up there in the choir front row was a man of principle and sturdy self-confidence, and could be calmly encouraging when my world seemed to be falling apart. Our love affair began that very first Sunday in church when we experienced a mind-boggling instant attraction. Later, just the sound of his voice on the phone saying my name would, as folks say, send me to Mars.

I was a young widow who had been hired by the senior rector to help with a clinical pastoral education program sponsored there. David occasionally dropped in at the office. His winning smile and peculiar work clothes had provoked enough curiosity that I, also a part-time columnist for a regional magazine, soon requested a personal interview about his family granite business. His grandfather had founded the Swenson Granite Company here in 1883. It is one of New Hampshire's many historic quarries. David had an extensive association with the company, dating back to being director beginning in 1961 and possessing vast knowledge of the business. I didn't know a thing about quarrying stone—its cutting, polishing, and finishing—and like most New Hampshire folk didn't know about the use of architectural stone in major public buildings nationwide, as in the CBS building in New York City, the Beinecke Rare Book & Manuscript Library at Yale, memorials such as the Tomb of the Unknown Soldier, and the Library of Congress. According to the *Concord Monitor* in 1999 the latter required three hundred men working six years to split and finish the 350,000 cubic feet of granite.

David's initial response that day to my request for an interview was to wear my boots. In the subsequent ride up Rattlesnake Hill in a very grimy gray Peugeot, I was aware of his exquisite manners and his Yale and Harvard education which transformed articulate knowledge of vague things like diamond saws into a fascinating encounter. Of course, I didn't hear a word he was explaining because I was wondering how any man could be that handsome and that smart at the same time.

". . . The flowers that bloom in the spring, tra la!" On that first tour of the quarry, we had discovered our jolly, mutual childhood memories of singing and dancing in Gilbert and Sullivan school productions. So he invited me to an operetta by chance being performed locally that week. My new presence in town evidently shocked his local Concord crowd when his friend Bert Whittemore, seated behind us, tapped me on the shoulder and bluntly asked "and who are *you*?"

Well, my identity has always been in question. From being an unwanted Melrose, Massachusetts child of the Depression years, to the child of a mother who demanded two hours of piano practice per day, to being a young pastor's wife back in the 1960s and 1970s in Ohio, Kentucky, Iowa, Connecticut, and Massachusetts (back when the churches got two for the price of one), to being a young widow, I had long wondered who I really was. (According to the Melrose High School yearbook, I was like a Powers' model, but most of all "reliable." Just what every girl wants to be called!) And Melrose was close enough to Boston to guarantee once-a-year kind of cultural exposure to the circus, the Ice Capades, and shopping in the original Filene's basement. Money was scarce, the idea of fun was illusive, and I had often lied to my parents that I didn't want things like a class ring or a Washington class trip when I really did. Summers in Bethel, Maine, with my grandparents simply highlighted my affinity for animals and blueberries, not people. My only brother, Walter, twelve years my senior, wrote "be moderate" in my little red autograph book. His advice sounded lofty but was totally irrelevant to my young thinking. My only sister, also years older, wore pretty heels and got married on a whirlwind weekend during World War II to her high school sweetheart, Roy.

As a pastor's wife (translate: an appendage), I once wrote only "Harriet" on my name tag. This lowly attempt at prime identity brought criticism and debate bordering on sacrilege. I still have trouble identifying myself on name tags. But being a mother to three sweet youngsters—Bill, Carolyn, and Laurie, was wonderful—I liked staying at home with them and listening to their dreams. Bill, a first rate juggler, wanted to be president; Carolyn worshipped Barbara Streisand's voice and the production of *Sound of Music*. Laurie wanted to be Mrs. Walton with at least eight children. Yet any dream of mine about being an independent, creative person, spontaneous and not bogged down by the limitations of the 1960s era view of marriage, just seemed beyond possibility—until, to combat the grief of my first husband's death, I switched from making some of our clothes to discovering the joy of turning scraps of colorful fabric into simple quilts through Church Women United projects. Only later, with David, my second husband, did I find a relief of feeling really known and loved for myself. He came from a well-respected family of means and reputation that included a younger brother, Malcolm, and his wife Barbara, and three children in Hanover; and an older brother, Guy (Andy), and his wife Mary, and three grown sons; along with two sisters, Betty and Mary Ellen and her husband, Bill, in Washington, DC, and their three grown children. David himself offered a degree of respect that I had seldom felt before, and exhibited a warm, loving role as uncle to his numerous nieces and nephews.

My lack of self-confidence had always troubled me, the self-deprecating opinion of myself probably lifelong. Life to my mother had seemed simply a strain. Her only real pleasures seemed to be Saturday afternoon operatic broadcasts, Saturday night Lawrence Welk concerts, and her hollyhocks, peonies, and bleeding hearts that grew beside our basement door. She couldn't understand why I didn't like clubby things such as Rainbow Girls and sororities, and worried a lot about what the neighbors would think about this or that. Well, I couldn't understand why she didn't like fantasy and spontaneous things. Five foot one in her Sunday hat (I'm five foot ten inches), she leaned on rules and naps and didn't know how to laugh. My father, six foot three, a silver-haired townie from Bethel, Maine, who had been valedictorian of Gould Academy, couldn't understand why his youngest daughter got As in everything but math. He was fond of the poem "Be the Best Little Tree." Denied any further education, he boarded the train for Boston and put himself through college. He loved chickens, Oldsmobiles, making fudge on Sunday afternoons, and smoking big stogies, and was known to stuff random bills into missionaries' pockets following a fiery sermon.

I connect many of my insecure fears to close watch by protective Victorian parents and an early marriage that meant trying to measure up to parishioner expectations in parsonage life. The system of changing pastorates could be grueling in a major Protestant denomination, and parsonage memories tend to stick. In Kentucky, with a student church, I had watched the delicious fried chicken served to males first. In Iowa, life had centered around many young gleeful children, and their periodic dramatic musical neighborhood productions were performed on our parsonage front porch. In Ohio, privacy didn't exist. With the parsonage smack up against the church building, we fielded phone calls day and night, interrupted by endless visits at both front and back doors. In Connecticut the train for New York City went through our backyard, and countless kittens were born in our bedroom closets. Everywhere, we were told never to establish friendships within the congregations because it stirred up petty jealousies.

Not knowing where our next ministry would be always took its toll. Obscure towns in obscure places; sparsely appointed parsonages with unmatched spigots and other people's furniture; seven-day weeks. Is it any wonder that later meeting and marrying a lovable middle-aged bachelor who shared my thirst for a plain home of our own felt like a miracle?

As the "good wife" I had always accompanied my first husband to job interviews. Wearing a weak smile and my one good dress, I would work hard at keeping silent about first impressions as the church and I checked each other out. The "call" was, of course, supposed to be coming from above. In reality, the decision depended on the quality of schools for our children, some prayer, good timing, and whether we "clicked" with the pulpit committee, who had their own tough job of picking a candidate out of the slush pile.

After my first husband's death from cancer at age forty-seven, and my years alone, life with passionate David in lovely New Hampshire was supposed to mean settling down at last in our own house with our own furniture with endless time for each other. Just to be accompanied by such a gentle, gracious, and undemanding person fulfilled me. He valued my opinion about things. His very smile warmed my being and promised a new look at living.

Our relationship began to appear serious to others when I had to again pass muster in the public eye when I was invited to meet his older brother, a Concord attorney.

II. Getting Acquainted

Yes, when I met his brother Andy that day, it felt like another test to see if I was good enough. But the Swensons did, in fact, welcome me, royally. Days became days and nights, sometimes tricky, as his friend Louis had to be ousted, and my daughter Carolyn—temporarily living with me—might pass him on the Contoocook road to Concord.

David and I soon found more and more ways, besides chance church encounters to be together. We played tennis (he was amazed at my backhand) and went sailing with friends in Portsmouth Harbor, where once a submarine surfaced nearby, creating a rather exhilarating response. We attended concerts at the Palace Theatre in Manchester, hosted lobster parties, and held hands in hidden moonlit places. There was always the rambling Swenson Beach House for a rendezvous. With its unique oceanfront setting, it was known to many, and was guaranteed to provide the laughter of somebody's children and the sound of raccoons scurrying within the walls. Jointly owned by five siblings, the house had three porches, eight bedrooms with dubious mattresses, a dining room the size of a dance hall, and a kitchen straight out of the dark ages. It was the only summer house on the point that boasted granite laundry posts because one summer, in a burst of energy, David had decided to replace the rotting wooden ones. In fact, David didn't do much resting during our allotted turn there. While most of us rushed to the waterfront, he was more apt to be heard saying, "I'm going to the hardware store." The truth is, the house was falling down.

Minor repairs were always needed, and major replacements were discussed over martinis. But we all loved the place, with its butler's pantry, giant linen closet, field-size parking lot, a strange little indoor elevator, and "our" bedroom in the back corner with its antique gray painted bedroom set. David always wanted the women to scour sinks and polish old lamp stands, but we thought food preparation was about all we could manage if we were *really* on vacation. He could count only on grandson Steve to take any interest in loading trash or grandson Ian to put the one air conditioner in or out.

There were endless overnight guests, parties, weddings, office retreats, and college reunions. So many people used the place that even with a schedule there were constant reminders: "don't leave us your dirty laundry again" or "For Pete's sake, don't forget that strange pudding in the refrig." But to everyone it was heaven in disguise.

Another favorite outing for us was traipsing to the annual League of New Hampshire Craftsmen show. Held in August at a scenic mountain near Lake Sunapee, it attracts thousands for the exhibition and sale. (During my stint with *New Hampshire Profiles* magazine, I had interviewed countless outstanding artists, with David and I liking the lively chats with them.) The sight of a CEO on vacation caught in mesmerized fascination with a skilled New Englander shaping a wrought iron gate or a classy ceramic pot brought us pleasure. The talent and the process and the philosophy of life was jointly appreciated. David and I had our own humble talents, but we were lifted up by its magnitude on display as we gobbled our picnic in folding chairs in the shade before dashing off for a dip in the lake.

Sunday afternoons became our favorite times together. Like two infatuated youngsters we would take off in his old Peugeot to explore the roads and towns of northern New Hampshire. With USGS maps stacked in back, and bathing suits thrown in the trunk, we did a bit of hiking but mostly a lot of wondrous getting to know each other.

From the beginning, and as experienced middle-agers, we had agreed on complete honesty, with no game playing in our new relationship. For both of us, middle age meant maturity derived from significant life experience. People make cracks about the sexuality attributed to older adults. You know those snickers on sitcoms. Well, our attraction was as hot and as physically expressive as that of any Hollywood teenager! I even told him I wasn't going back to the kitchen (church suppers were a nightmare for me), to which he had said "Don't worry. We'll eat out." I thought that was generous of him, considering he'd been eating out most of his single adult life. Of course, I knew that really wasn't going to happen. But, it was enough that this wonderful fellow really loved *me*.

David, comfortable and confident in his blue ribbon identity, and seldom downhearted, had endured endless efforts to be paired off with somebody's sister or cousin. To his embarrassment, he had often been introduced by his father as "my son who never married." He had wanted to be a farmer but ended up at Yale and Harvard. (His IQ was scary; I was told that during wartime he had gotten such a high test score that he was actually put in charge of a troop train as a young recruit and assigned to intelligence!) He was probably one of those annoying smart kids who got top grades without any effort. His parents' expectation of him was high but relaxed; in fact when his father had dropped him off at Phillips Academy Andover, he simply turned in his seat and said, "It's your life now" and drove off.

Perhaps farming seemed a way of life that promised to be carefree, or it promised a chance for casual dressing. Everyone, it seems, knew that David cared little about his attire. (I eventually gave up on bringing home stylish clothing suggestions or updated matches.) He thought that money spent on clothes was wasted money, yet he repeatedly told me, "I like the way *you* dress!" The truth is, when David chose to spruce himself up, he was a knockout, even though the outfit might be more than twenty-five years old or had been part of a certain now dead Mr. Jenkins' hand-me-down wardrobe.

From the start I had liked so many things about him. He had eyes like George Clooney, was considered an Omar Sharif look-alike, and, according to his niece Iwonka, was a "dashingly handsome man, Cary Grant handsome!" David's quiet manner and dry sense of humor were admirable, too, but I admit it was his welcome tendency to help with the dinner dishes that sealed our relationship.

After finding pleasure hand cutting paving blocks with former Concord Police Chief Walt Carlson, David liked to define himself as a "plodder"—a word often stated in derision. The fact is that many of David's bachelor days were highlighted by meals at the Archway Restaurant, with Barb and Ernie recommending the shrimp specialty over, say, the lamb shank, his drink at the ready, and that for five long years he cared for his bedridden father. A plodder may not be written up in academic journals or social pages, but he takes time to converse with plumbers as well as presidents and is often remembered regardless of what he is wearing. When David wore his ancient Brooks Brothers white summer slacks with the "hand wash separately"label, the slight yellowing at the knee had made little difference to him. When he wore them last, he was probably asking about somebody's grandchild.

I had begun to realize how the word "granite" was splashed all over the state, a popular choice of name for stores, utilities, and sports teams, and I learned there had once been forty-four quarries in the area. Actually, my introduction to the world of stone began on those first Sunday afternoons of countryside exploration when David would suddenly stop the car and declare, "Look at that!"

"What?"

Puzzled, I would blindly gaze in various directions, seeing nothing in particular.

"That basement foundation is from . . ."

"Those front steps are from Georgia."

Or sometimes on a rural back road we would come to an abrupt halt near a picturesque cemetery, and he would point out a gracefully carved angel on a headstone. "Oh, those Italian craftsmen are *so* gifted." Or there would be a very humble design on a colonial gravestone with a unique engraving, or a gatepost that seemed to have stepped out of Versailles in its gracefulness.

So I learned some New Hampshire history about stone. How the early settlers cleared the many rocks to make room for planting; how the uses of granite went from dark basement foundations to durable widespread exterior use in public buildings to the curbing of large and small highways, to diversified products for industries and personal home use, as in gardens. And according to the company's current chairman, cousin Kurt Swenson, I learned that the John Swenson Granite Company had been a leader in worker safety, his great-grandfather's company the first in granite in the United States to install dust collection equipment to eliminate the risk of silicosis.

I got used to the subject after a while, and soon realized that a quick stop meant that a curbstone workman was going to get free advice about setting a stone. And I became increasingly impressed by the vast variety of stone colorations and spectacular hues from around the world, now displayed in showrooms, as granite grew in popularity for use in kitchens and bathrooms.

Everyone was becoming an overnight connoisseur, but David's ability to quickly identify a particular stone from a moving distance always startled me and was more impressive than his geology degree or his Harvard MBA.

So I joined the reverence.

We marveled at our own similarities. He liked to hand-cut and set paving blocks, and I liked to cut and sew quilting blocks. (Did we both have some sort of mindset about order and precision?) We had sisters with similar names—Mary Ella and Mary Ellen. (Sadly, his sister passed soon after we married.) We both had rather strange preferences in music. It was Gilbert and Sullivan and opera. (Most of the time the latter was too pricey for our frugal habits.) Neither of us had been allowed to have animals as children. It was my sister, commuting from Boston, who finally defied my mother and via the train brought home a cat in a shoebox.

Growing up I had loved other people's pets and regularly took my young children to visit the local SPCA and tried not to bring home the dog that smiled at me. (There had been many dogs in our parsonage homes: the Samoyed who bit the mailman, the black Labrador retriever who got hit by a car, the beagle who chewed dollar bills, the golden retriever who chased neighbor's chickens, the Irish setter who jumped out a window, the German shepherd who didn't like wiggly children, the collie who preferred to sit in her wing chair by the picture window.) Owning various four-footed creatures brought more love to my makeshift parsonage homes. So then there was David's dog, Cecil. David as a child had never gotten over the pet goat next door being killed and served up on a platter for his neighbor's dinner. Cecil, his first dog, became his dutiful companion and part of our happy home for many years.

You could say that the plodder and the reliable Powers model almost became one. As for our differences, there were, of course, a few. While I was quick to define similarities, I can now be more factual. He balanced checkbooks to the penny while I rounded everything off. We cancelled each others' votes in political contests. His love of human nature, in contrast to my skeptical view, can be illustrated in his abrupt stopping in the midst of a busy London airport to exclaim, "Good grief, I ought to know one person in this giant crowd!" This still brings a chuckle. Politics were seldom mentioned with the Swenson clan because heated representation of all viewpoints was guaranteed.

When traveling, David would carry a large briefcase with a toothbrush and a change of underwear and would whistle his way out the door to a business trip. I worried about every detail. I carried one light suitcase and kept track of traveler's checks and peculiar pocket change. He never worried about the exchange rate or any language problem, and he found all people terribly interesting. The global network was intriguing to him, not threatening, whether in business or pleasure. He never complained of my lack of expertise; we just witnessed all the beauty or novelty together.

He showed me Paris, Italy, Sweden, and Portugal, and the artistic ambiance of Florence became embedded in my soul forever. In turn, he actually loved it when I showed him the tamer highlights of Kentucky—Calumet Downs, the Berea Arts Festival, Thomas Merton's monastery, Coach Rupp's territory, and of course New Hampshire's Star Island on the Isles of Shoals.

Oh, the memories. Tears still come to my eyes on mere remembrance of our wedding! "Oh ring the merry bells on board ship!"

III. Bliss

We had decided on February for the big day, as, according to David, that was a slow time for the stone business. In our preference for simplicity and frugality, we then hired a talented calligrapher to design our modest invitation—elegant script on an oversized soft gray index card, with David, on noting the need for color, hand painting the single rose on each invitation. Likewise, in our non-conventional mode, we added "no gifts, please." (We had two houses to sell and no need of additional toasters.) Then David accompanied me on the train to Boston as I shopped for a wedding dress. (The trip actually inspired me to design and make my own— wool, of course as winter in New Hampshire is notoriously cold.) There were festive showers and a dinner party sponsored by many Swensons who appeared from far and near to celebrate, with many folks remarking that they had never seen David so happy. (His grabbing me and kissing me in public view provided novel entertainment for both reticent family observer and stranger.)

The traditional ceremony, was, of course, held at St. Paul's Episcopal Church in Concord with David's niece Iwonka our flower girl and Ian, my five-year-old grandson, our ring bearer. The reception was held at the Society for the Protection of New Hampshire Forests, an award-winning building within the Concord city limits. I had made all the royal blue tablecloths for the informal reception, and we went off to Eleuthera, an island in the Bahamas. Our romantic honeymoon cottage provided lots of time to digest the immeasurable joy of nonstop togetherness before returning to our quaint old Cape Cod style house in Canterbury, New Hampshire which was to be our temporary home.

Our search for simplicity had led us to this small Shaker town, ten miles from Concord, where we soon became active members of the small community church, the annual July 31, fair and the annual Gilbert and Sullivan production with its endless rehearsals and rollicking cast parties. Its handy village store and post office, with its promise of daily friendly greetings, and its ancient cemetery added to the ambiance. Then there was the fascinating Shaker history, and quaint buildings, lilting music, and stories about early residents who had taken in orphans and invented things like brooms and cloaks and pincushions. The very air seemed to inspire me as I designed fabricated wall hangings for the McGowan Art Gallery, designed costumes for our Gilbert and Sullivan productions, and wrote a meditation book based on quilting. I accompanied David on occasional business trips and to local festivities such as Fifield family ice cutting parties in town. I went back to school for a master's degree, finding energy to commute to Boston.

Our temporary move, which included the addition of a romantic bedroom overlooking a new screened porch and an iris garden, became an eight-year stay because we loved our time together there so much. During this enchanted stay, Bill and Carolyn graduated from college and Laurie and her husband, Rick, produced four more beautiful grandchildren—Steve, Kayley, Leah, and Jayne—to join young Ian.

But after years scouting out an inexpensive house on the coast of New England, we finally found a nice old Durham New Englander that had been somewhat destroyed by college students who had rented rooms there. Ten minutes from historic Portsmouth and on the outskirts of a university town, our dream house had brought comments like "Why did you buy that thing?" because we had to remove a raunchy apartment, linoleum that had never been tacked down, and a refrigerator in the living room. But we saw its alluring potential with its hillside view sloping down to and across Route 4 to the bay. So we joyfully went to work. I painted the front door Venetian rose, bought high-standing bookshelves, and actually thought it was fun to paint and paper because I had done it on all those old parsonages in my earlier life. But this house was ours and special. There was space for two offices, and David found special pleasure each Christmas by wrapping garlands around the front porch columns and placing a floodlight on the five-foot wreath on the attached shed near the back entry.

Although the quaint old farmhouse needed significant work, we did not worry about rushing to get things done. We didn't allow even a loose door handle to upset us. It was a stressless daily routine that included the spirit of adventure. It was the beginning of an era of being relaxed and balanced, of letting go of the past, without pressure to seek endless perfection. We had settled in forever. We simply delighted in the project—an occasional update, finding meaning in the blessing of a side-by-side endeavor after our extended years of living alone. We repaired what was necessary, with plumbers and carpenters making occasional visits, and lived without cultural standards dictating our efforts. We planted a few flowers, hooked up a dog run, and added a granite post for the mailbox. We were of course always frugal to the core, sometimes hiring special help if needed but able to postpone and procrastinate like everyone else. We ordered an enchanting old rose carpet runner for the front stairway. If the forecast was for light snow, we simply settled in for a cozy rendezvous. If the sun was shining, we often drove up the Maine coast to view York Beach, the Nubble Light, and Marginal Way, or wound around the rockbound coast by the Bush compound. Sometimes we would rake a few leaves or smell the lilacs, cutting short the effort if we thought about the salad bar or fish dinners at Warren's Lobster House in Kittery.

David introduced me to his many friends, mostly from Concord days, which brought me to learn about Buzz's camp or Tom's boat, those friendships forged by privileged childhoods. These informal friends, and often witty, and having chosen to retire in New Hampshire, provided warmth and meaning to our lives.

It was a contented way of living. I felt greeted each day by hope and possibility. I didn't let questions and uncertainty rule. Perhaps the sense of fullness was brought on by the big old house with high ceilings and tall windows, being near the exuberance of university students (who think it's warm enough for shorts when the temperature rises to thirty-two degrees.) We were also near the many special events at the Whittemore Center; the extensive University of New Hampshire library; historic Portsmouth, with its rapidly expanding coastal ambiance; the Portsmouth Naval Shipyard; and the buzz of Pease Air Force Base. Even Cecil joined us in our car or giant yard, frolicking happily while obeying David's unique manner of instruction—swinging his arm in a chosen direction, not yelling impatient orders or demands. Summers meant being close enough to the beach house to visit with the many Swenson relatives who took their turns at residence each year come summer.

This move to the coast included the choice of First Parish Church in Dover as our church affiliation. After a year of visiting several churches in the area with David, he had insisted that I be the one to choose a church home. This was not easy. Both of us had been raised by parents who expected church attendance, and we found inspiration in many places, often based on exceptional musical programming. We became regular members and supported many programs, and I served on the diaconate and renovation committee of this large downtown place of worship.

Life had in many ways opened up for me as certain old disturbing memories slipped away. I had allowed people to dictate my life because my sense of self had been so small. I had seldom voiced rebellion or declared rights or, as folks say today, "processed it" because I did not know how. My life had run according to authority figures who seldom asked about my wishes.

I had once been bedridden for three months without nursing care then had gone into labor while alone and watching my three preschool-age children.

The poverty and peculiarities of being in the ministry in the 1950s and 1960s had deeply affected my approach to all of life. Parsonage life as it was once lived by clergy families was seldom understood by the average churchgoer. (According to my sister, my grandfather Clark sat down and cried when he learned that little Harriet was going to marry a minister.) The ways things were, however, does not downgrade the membership of those pastorates. There were always wonderful folks who tried to live decent lives as they saw it. But life in a fishbowl was often debilitating. Life for our family was so focused on church affairs that we once tried fining all family members five cents if they mentioned the church during dinner.

From the outside, it appeared to be a free ride for the pastor and his family, but in reality it was anything but. The church provided housing as part of a benefits package, but there was a trade-off. The chance to invest in a modest house that would later provide housing for retirement living was generally not allowed. Today, many protestant church leaders—male and female—finance their own housing arrangements. Moreover, in those days, the wife was supposed to work, gratis, at home and church, a separate career unthinkable. Being the preacher's wife had represented an identity that I allowed to be "enough," so I am to blame for not trying to find out who I was meant to be. There was a falseness to it—to just smile and let hubby lead the way, to be subservient to the status quo.

Those early years in the pastorate with my first husband were hectic, frugal, and demanding—and singularly memorable. My then husband and I found that the youthful call to try to save the world could feed despair. Much was done out of duty, but we both learned basics about human nature, along with the absurd, the distinguishing, the catastrophic, and the humble and inspiring. The lack of flush toilets was nothing compared to the heart-wrenching family secrets revealed to me, the minister's wife, over a large sink full of dishes. My world felt like a wide-mouthed thermos, gasping for more, always wanting more than I seemed able to contribute.

At age twenty I had left college to support my first husband's seminary education. We lived in one-room apartments and then modest parsonages. Twenty years later when I was able to enroll in college to finish a degree, he was diagnosed with lung cancer while senior minister of the picturesque Lynnfield, Massachusetts,

Congregational church. His words "You're going to drop out, of course" were answered with a resounding "No! How else will I support our children?" And I proceeded to take CLEP (College Level Examination Program) exams, win a Clairol scholarship and graduate soon after his death.

When I later moved to New Hampshire to be near my sister and be away from the town where it looked as though my identity would always be "that preacher's widow," I had questions, some of them stupid, such as "Will God still love me if I don't go to church on Sunday?" Solemn memories of a churchy childhood kept popping into my head at strange times, as in the childhood highlight of winning a box of cornflakes at a church raffle, only to have it taken back because I was not an adult and was not meant to win, or in the bribe of peppermints or a piece of gum to keep me sitting still during the endless morning service. Or the scripture verses memorized or the haunting melodies from hymns hummed accidentally. Surprisingly, I would later find I liked the ritual of the Episcopal Church where I was employed. Would Gilbert and Sullivan say I was again breaking rank?

Having once rushed into an early marriage, I wasn't going to do that again. After moving to New Hampshire as a widow, I was simply finding immense pleasure checking out Sunday morning flea markets in my comfortable old clothes (another similarity to David's lifestyle) as I considered running an antiques shop out of my barn, not to mention that I had always felt cheated out of weekend excitement. I had been raised to believe that young girls could not shop or wear sport clothes on Sunday, the afternoon thus becoming long and boring while friends could play outside and roller skate and shout, and I could only hide in the bedroom to listen to *The Shadow* on the radio.

So when David was diagnosed and we saw our newfound dreams of continued bliss evaporate, all afternoons and evenings and mornings, all twenty-four-hour days, took on new face masks.

IV. Trouble

After those wonderful years with David in Canterbury and Durham, he began to have breathing difficulties. The shock of sickness and uncertainty with its many kinds of ugly questions began to drown out the idyllic life of love and sharing we had been living. After at last finding someone so magically compatible, would he be taken away? The treadmill of time to be unchosen, cut short? His former smoking habit, combined with stone dust and asthma, had eventually led to a diagnosis of COPD (chronic obstructive pulmonary disease) and small cell lung cancer, beginning a six-year rigid regimen of different inhalers, a gradual shift from nighttime to full-time oxygen, many medications and rounds of chemotherapy and radiation, and a total change in how we would live out what was left of our daily survival in Camelot.

Panic began to take over. Worst of all would be the wretched pain of again watching another loved one struggle and die, not to mention the old fears of being left with limited funds, endless paperwork, oceans of pity, and especially the worry over the future for Bill, Carolyn, and Laurie.

I should begin by explaining that I tend to wince in terror at anything medical. Perhaps it is because in my family of origin we leaned toward an artistic rather than a scientific mentality. Perhaps, too, it was being raised by a sickly mother who was not emotionally available to me as a teen. For whatever reason, it took a while for David and me to find our own voices within the complex medical system.

Yes, the children were grown this time, as death again hovered, and as fear and intimidation with questions silently surfaced and nagged. On those first days of shock after the diagnosis, the raw data jumped out at me at the doctor's office: the picture of the large crimson and pink cross-section of the human circulatory system posed immodestly on a medical office wall. We, the paper poster and I, would stare at each other before I turned away. The realization that there can be deadly bright red antibodies traveling the highways of David's invisible places felt suspicious, too horribly familiar. David, David I had always liked green better anyway. Green promises sunlight and growth and flowers and, as the poet says, "new blossoms of me," so to escape I often envisioned a certain quilt pattern done in shades of emerald and rose, almost soothing and fragrant.

We forget our questions for the doctor. We declare we won't come in again until we are addressed by our last, not first names.

We are told to make lists of concerns. It is so easy to blame someone else.

I was racked with remembrance of my first husband's death; scenes from the past continued to haunt me, darting on and off the screen of consciousness: all those trips to the hospital for painful draining of his lungs, the fact that I could not give injections, the time I was not strong enough to lift him out of the bathtub, the process of begging the Massachusetts General Hospital bigwig medical man to release him long enough for me to drive him to the Portsmouth ferry to go out to the Shoals to say good-bye to our summer friends, to wrestle a wheelchair on and off the boat.

How could I do this *again*? Fury, with its unfair rage and panic, took over. Gritting my teeth, I reviewed the basic facts of my second marriage.

Granite business is cyclical, and, according to David, managing a stone company can mean turning one's salary back into the company if there is a downswing. No longer associated with the company, David was paying all his drug bills out of pocket, and he had no pension. And we were certainly both familiar with hand-me-down outfits. But I was not just thinking of being frugal; I became really terrified. I was remembering. I had seen, firsthand, many faces of poverty, including my own. A distant memory of "Where'ere You Walk," being sung by my first husband to my accompaniment on our old black upright in an Iowa back room, surfaced from somewhere to keep me focused.

In the beginning, facing another fearful approach of death, and loss, it was logical that solitary walking became my momentary escape. (As a kid I had walked three miles to high school and three miles back.) So I walked in the morning with the young mothers in the Durham neighborhood who had just placed their kids on the school bus. They were such good company, and they walked with energy and fire as well as kindness. I even dared to share what I knew about walking. Prayer walking can be done anywhere, indoors or out. Linus Mundy's book about it gives excellent suggestions for short, thoughtful phrases that have a beat. Labyrinth walking based on a thirteenth-century custom that involves following an ancient circular floor pattern as a metaphor for centering life. Escape walking: Rousseau said that one just goes out and discovers that plain walking stimulates the mind while Thoreau said the best is done with an attitude of sauntering rather than purpose.

So walking provided a good time to again weigh options, make hard decisions.

The idea of quietly walking beside a loved one during illness may seem idiotic in a world with ballistic missile systems, powerful SUV vehicles, and orbiting satellites. It was not easy to deliberately tune out the steady background of grinding cultural chatter. Later, when I took a walk along a coastal beach, I again tried to hash things over, my mind unable to accept the truth about David's illness. Lung surgery not possible. Would he eventually suffer the horrors of suffocation, experience total dependency on respirator care? Dear God, NO!

The houses on Wells Beach, Maine, on that first runawayday reminded me of people's faces. Walking the large curved beachfront off season, I mulled over the row of silent cottages, seeing them as ordinary folks. They, like us, displayed silent utterings: cared for, forgotten, fixed up, barely surviving, just pretending, and all facing the same direction in a frozen stance of avid listening. Yet they were starkly diversified. Gray, summer white, mottled green. Windows large, too small, peculiar, broken, cleverly renovated, all in houses of vastly different architectural styles: trendy, spacious, traditional, simple. Attempts at grand; success at neglect.

Together, midwinter, strung on a necklace of uncertainty, they were silent, but their outward appearance declared a lot about identity, worries about tomorrow, and plain survival, looking out to unlimited horizons for any helpful messages.

I was one of those boarded-up houses.

How could I become the strong kind of caregiver needed?

I needed a rock, or at least a cobblestone. My spirit and lifelong habits were monogrammed only with oughts. So with David's illness had come more deep, unresolved questions. Faith and hope were a blur of stamina and panic.

I had been subservient to orthodoxy until summertime conferences and cherry picking into philosophy and literature. Then various other influences had come my way: an advanced degree in research at an accredited seminary, an earlier job with a major publishing company, a fascination with Eastern philosophy, a release from the pious literal of the political arena, the bravery of peers who explored things that their parents hadn't allowed, the realization that God could be a woman.

Everyone has a story, and mine, beneath the rage and frustration, was slowly unfolding to me. There was no denominational ploy or pious orthodoxy here, but there was a frank new view within my generation when caught in certain long-held attitudes about illness and death and life and the medical world in which we now live. Sickness could change everything.

I did not know what to do with those raging feelings about what could be a terminal condition and my impending loss of a devoted husband. I found myself harboring garbled thoughts that needed to be glued down or confronted. Maybe write things down? Maybe tame the anger and frustration? For example, it is assumed that all women are automatic caregivers. Well, regardless of degree of love and devotion, we sometimes are not, and I soon found myself writing down random thoughts about our new daily routines, raggedly incomplete, so filled with anguish of the moment, revealing only a fluctuating state of mind as a wild mix of new questions salted the daily coping and flooded the day.

Is my rage so explosive that it could become offensive? Will it go away if I admit certain feelings? Do I think that mere thoughts could eventually become a best seller? Or puzzling questions, such as: What do I know about caregiving? How could I live without David? What will give me the ability/strength to carry on?

Having also been a magazine columnist, I began to consider capturing the essence of a home caregiver's life in a way that could be passed on to others. I dreamed of taking my frantic scribbles and translating them into a lively roller coaster ride of blunt observations, mood swings, places of solace, and poetic grieving that had become my caregiver's entire life. What was for me a short therapeutic account could, I hope, be for the unprepared caregiving reader a revelatory window—from lyrical to practical, from maudlin to philosophical, and probably some of the very same things other caregivers sought, except that desperately loving someone who needs your undivided attention is unlike anything else. Maybe I would separate the caregiving years into a special section of the frustrated loving and who I was or had to be, before and after he left me. There are a lot of maybes in life!

Much later, before I again stepped on board the Thomas Laighton ferry in Portsmouth Harbor to head out to Star Island, I would also feel a strange urge to scribble down two other flaming words—"flogged identity"—on a scrap of paper in the kitchen, not really knowing how that phrase applied to me. Flogged? To be beaten with a stick? No. I had been raised in a typical New England family, provided with basic necessities, but had gone on to live in two extreme worlds: from tilting outhouses in rural Kentucky to prosperous coastal towns with five-car garages in New England.

So scraps of paper and small notebooks sprouted here and there around our honeymoon house and around our leased car. Litter accumulated as both poetic and gunpowder outbursts on the backs of things—random words and phrases of real-life experience to organize and edit. Mood swings, private thoughts, small luxuries: ideas took shape. Could I expand each thought into a daily reading? So I soon toted home some large yellow legal pads of paper. Both a relief and a curse, the single words and phrases of my turned-around life began to grow into readable passages.

I guess faith falters and forges ahead under the worst and best of circumstances. The journey of life and death has been told in many ways, but what finally became my humble offering here is unique. After David's death, the final account is written from *my* perspective as home caregiver, not that of the patient, loving though the relationship was. My saga is true, told through the daily mundane events of sickness and surviving. And maybe it could be healing for not only myself but for families also giving it. Then again, maybe the idea is crazy. Maybe I do bond only with animals!

As I began to acknowledge the fullness of what became middle-age, I decided that falling in love again at age fifty-one had changed my entire life. I was not just a little ol' lady who had a love affair. He had not been just a New Hampshire lad who wore plaid flannel shirts and as a Harvard MBA calmly balanced his checkbook to the penny.

When two people like us find each other, everything explodes. To believe you are a person of value is fundamental. To know that your individual life can have meaning turns everything around. Snicker and flap may abound in our culture when elders mention the power of their newfound love, but many of us elders, products of a new breed of age bracket, know the truth. David had loved me for who I was. I had loved David for who he was. When he died, who I seemed to be staggered around for a while, but I did survive and had a new perspective from the pain and loss. What changed for me? I don't know how to best describe it. Perhaps it was really David who was the teacher, who provided strength for us both and gave me courage to carry on.

From frugality to fear to freedom to everlasting love?

For now let me tell you what the six-year role of caregiver felt like with David through the following short, finally finished daily readings, along with a few observations about grief and gratitude and a woman's life that continues on and on. Walk with me as I think out loud, and let it all hang out. See what mysteriously emerges in the gradual foggy return to everydays. Step back in time with me. Maybe I was just talking to myself when I wrote these, but real love made such a difference.

The death of a lover is a path, said Ram Dass.

THE CAREGIVING YEARS

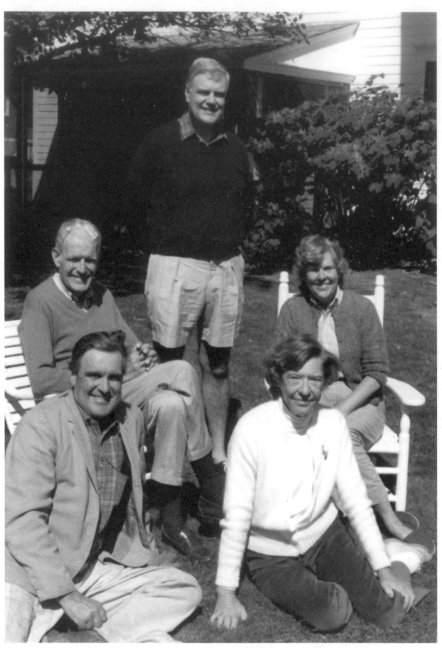

David (on grass) and his siblings: Malcolm Swenson (top), Betty (seated right), Mary Ellen (on grass), and Guy (seated left).

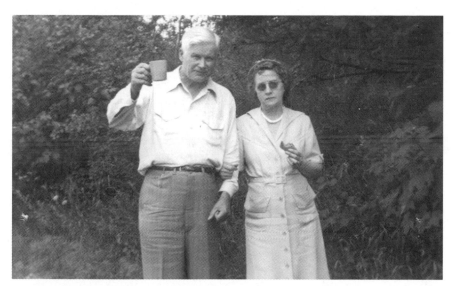

My parents on another picnic.

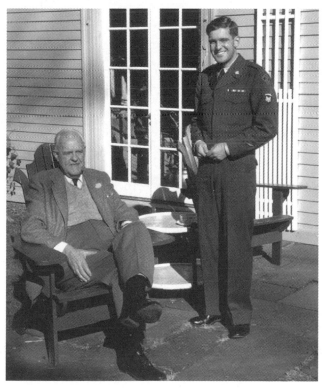

Father and son.

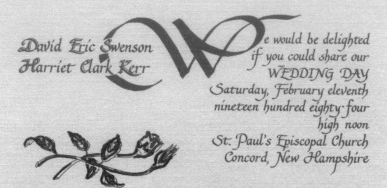

Wedding invitation.

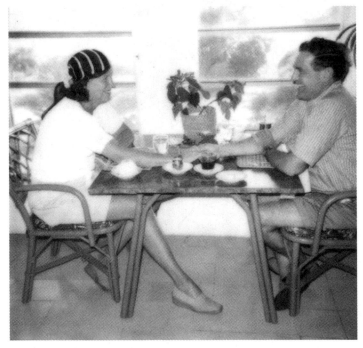

Eleuthera bliss.

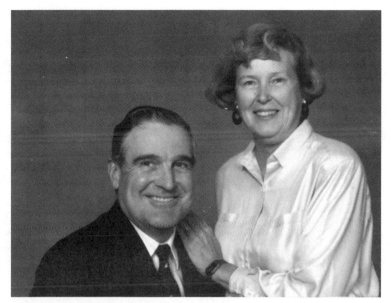

Church directory pose.

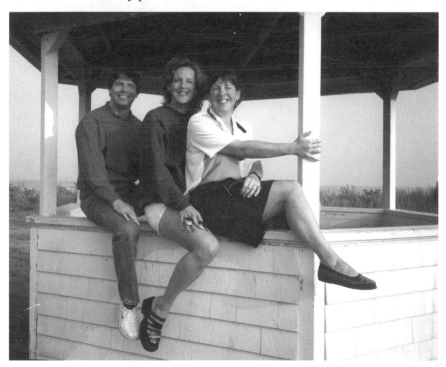

My children: Bill, Carolyn, Laurie.

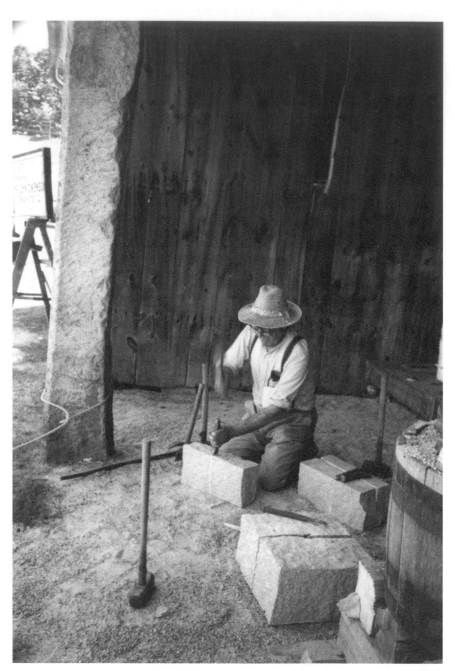

David's favorite past-time (cutting stone).

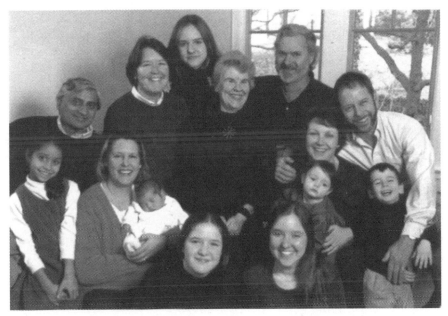

Some of the Washington DC Swensons.

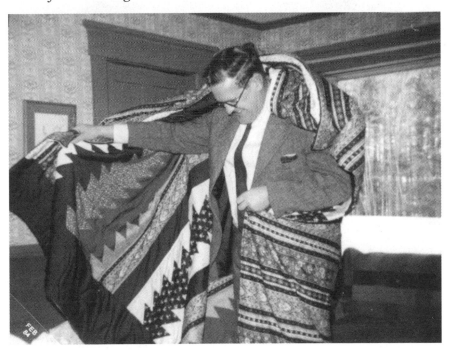

David admires my work.

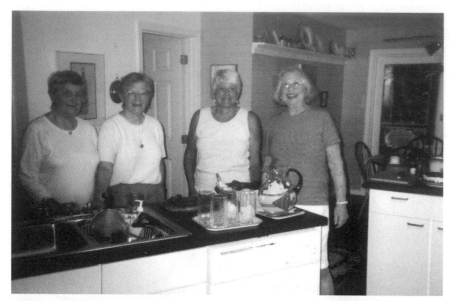

My monthly discussion group; haven of support.

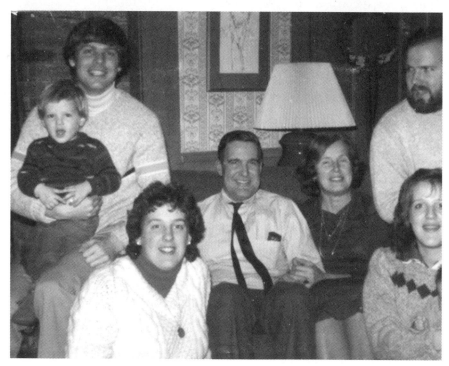

Creation of a new family.

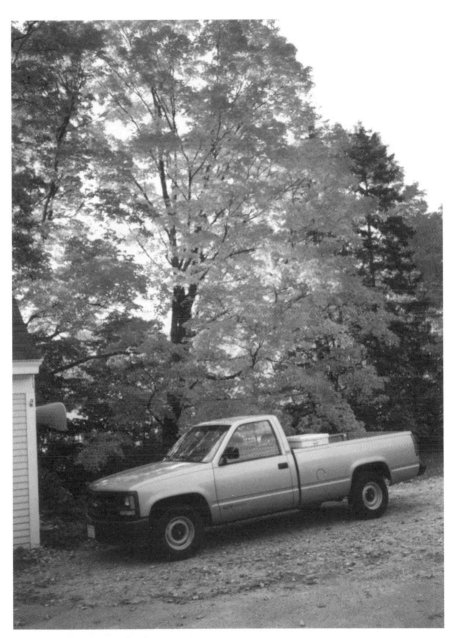

David's favorite vehicle.

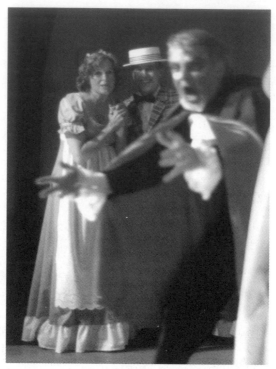

Harriet and David in Canterbury
Gilbert & Sullivan production.

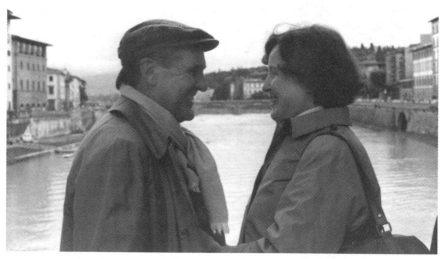

Harriet and David in Italy.

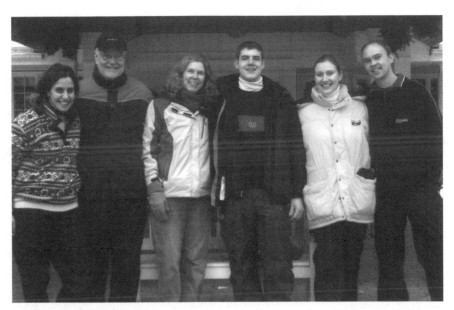

Malcolm's family.

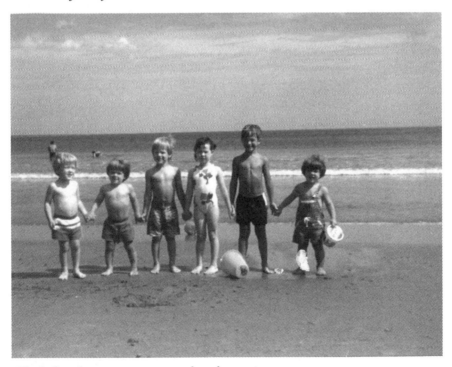

Clark family cousins swim at beach reunion.

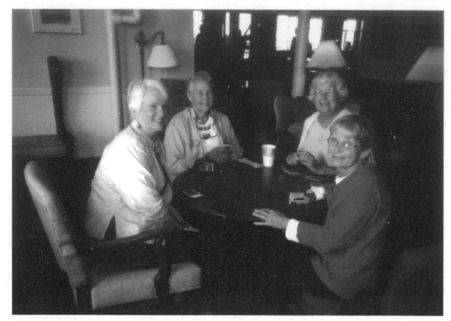

Relaxing bridge game at Star.

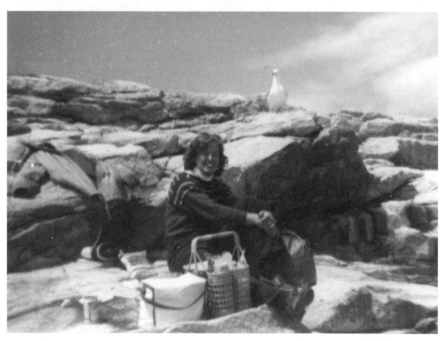

Our first Star Island picnic.

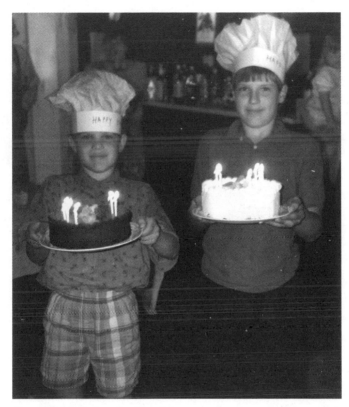

Special birthday for David.

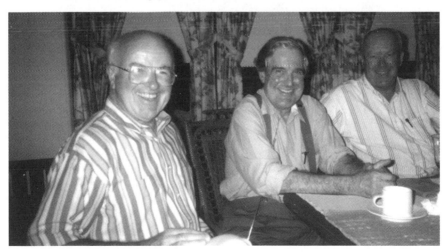

Three longtime Concord buddies.

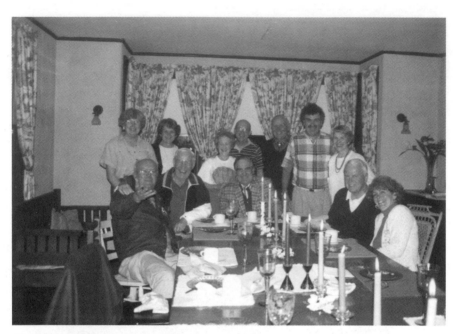

Beach house lobster party.

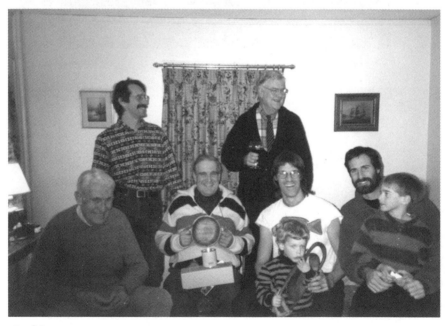

Andy's sons come visiting.

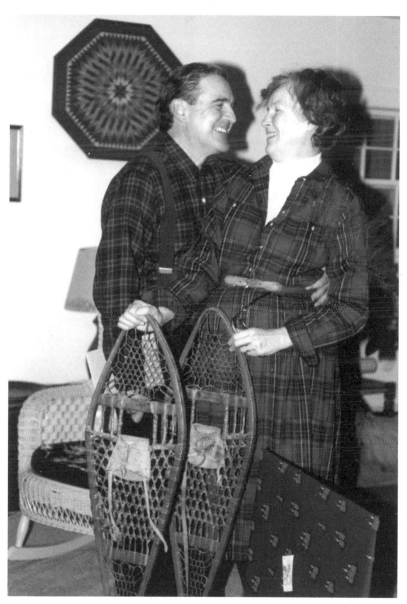

Winter in New Hampshire.

V. Daily Thoughts

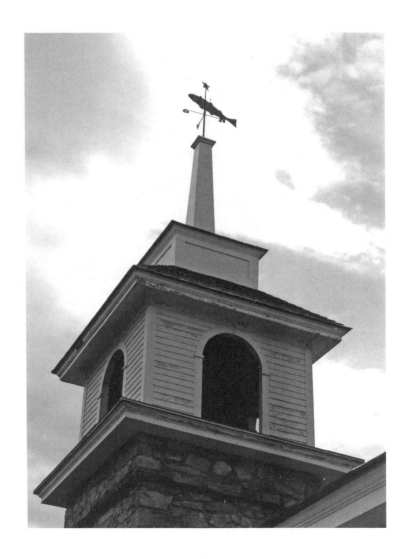

WAITING ROOM

Find two seats.

Again we sit in the waiting area of the cancer center. The battlefield always the same, our headquarters ruled by a close regiment of chairs, steel blue in color, that soldier walls adorned with innocuous prints done in sickly pastels.

We know the drill. To wait, mute, for top brass orders.

A soft whish on our right heralds the opening of the automatic entry gate. This ushers in another unwilling recruit while the dreary gray commercial carpet does its best to hide the sound of his slow, hesitant shuffling entrance.

Worn magazines and game books scattered on low tables supply some distraction; an unfinished jigsaw puzzle depicting a remote English cottage has been worked on by shaking hands. A chatty fellow in a Bull's cap now dares to get up to stagger crosswise for a child-size taste of water, and all eyes, wary, synchronize his ambling forward and back to the beat of a rabid TV host ranting loudly about nonessentials.

Enter the sentinel of hope, a uniformed nurse calling out dubiously, "David Swenson?" Armored in Nikes and a crooked name tag sagging on a limp string, she coolly fans out her search. Jarred to attention, our emotions compressed, we scramble up, daring to follow.

FRIENDSHIP

The offer by phone saying "I think it's something you'll like" feels generous. A friend is taking time in her busy day to drive over and hand me a paperback, *Modoc*. A book about an elephant.

I am at first dubious.

Mysteries for escape or biographies of enchanting twelfth-century mystics have more initial appeal to me. So the book sits by my comfy pink chair while I finish a thriller by P. D. James. But a glimpse of a real child's attachment to a circus elephant and the kind of lasting relationship that develops through very difficult years keeps me enthralled in whatever spare moment I can muster.

My friend knows me, I conclude upon finishing the delightful tale. She knows I love animals. Knew I would love this book. Her kindness relieves the moment.

LOST

David and I have been so fortunate, to date. We live in a land of boat-cover blue and stubborn but humorous provincialism adjacent to lakes and mountains with enchanting Indian names like Wanalancet, Contoocook, and Piscataqua. Like the hoards of tourists who prowl our magnificent terrain, we, too, at times get lost.

I will never forget the time David decided to scout out Mount Agamenticus. He assumed it was just a short detour from Route 1 on which we were headed home.

It was dusk, and the winding roads were not giving up proper signs. Although the gas gauge was almost on empty, David was determined to find the modest mountain. We headed for home via the correct compass direction, coasting as much as possible on a road that was wildly unfamiliar. I was frightened beyond words, knowing that with David's breathing condition any emergency decision would be up to me. A familiar landmark provided direction and a topic of conversation for the future.

In the meantime we were lost.

But now I feel lost again. Another back road? Who will fix this?

New Englanders have always been known for surprises. The repairman who once came to check the furnace fixed the doorbell; later, when we called the electrician to fix the closet light, he put up our Christmas tree.

We prefer to rely on ourselves, but sickness means cruising the possibilities.

QUARTERS

We save quarters for Leah, our granddaughter. (We have five grand-children from my first marriage.) The new kind of coin is now issued in groups of four U.S. states per year. I just got Louisiana today! We had even bought the large cardboard map of the United States with its punched-out places for the shiny new pictorial change. When I say to a store clerk, "You can't have that one!" she patiently checks for others and we trade, big-time.

Collecting quarters seems like such a luxury. Pennies in a jar were once the fashion, and it took forever to hoard enough to buy a book or a bracelet. I think things have gone up.

My father arose each morning and cackled pleasantly that it was "another day, another dollar." Now I get up, stressed, and wonder where I am going to park if I go to town. Parking at the UNH library lot means twenty-five cents per fifteen minutes, and parking in down-town Portsmouth means circling three times and settling on a place where a ticket is imminent if I'm caught or unable to figure out that new kind of meter.

Just what do coins buy now besides memories? A quarter-pounder has little to do with five nickels or twenty-five pennies, and a quarter of a lifetime suggests something in four parts, with David and I embarking on the last segment, supposedly called golden.

Priceless, yes, but condemning us to brace for separation.

CECIL

We pretend that our lives are normal, that nothing has changed. We eat three meals a day, attend church, and practice our regular New Hampshire frugality by proceeding with our renovation of "this old house."

We continue to take Cecil who sits proudly in the Dodge truck as we drive to Wagon Hill Farm, where joggers, dog lovers, and picnic enthusiasts amble over five hundred acres by Great Bay. Cecil is David's first dog, a large mongrel Rhodesian Ridgeback who seldom lets David out of his sight. Ten years of front-seat sitting in the old blue pickup makes this a familiar outing. On approaching the park entrance, Cecil throws back his head to howl in joyful anticipation of again running free. On Tuesdays and Thursdays he accompanies David to rehab. Even at his advanced dog age, he retains, come summer, a nomadic gypsy spirit as he runs off to the salt marshes with his wagging friends.

When neurological problems cause Cecil's hind legs to fail, I learn to dress him in dog booties three times a day before he drags his hind feet down into the field for relief. He continues to sleep in our room beneath our open bedroom window, where he sometimes roars up to a sudden alert when the odor of coyote dares to drift in.

So together David and I practice elementary caregiving, not dreaming that it is comparable in some ways to a human rehearsal.

BROCHURES

I sit in a hospital waiting room again.

I ponder the titles of the endless pamphlets and brochures tucked into a large wall display board, and hope for the colorful photographic flashes of tourist ads about our scenic New Hampshire. Instead I see Having a Pelvic Exam, Sail Through Surgery, About Smoking, Massage Therapy, Testicular Self-Examination, What You Need to Know About.

The intent of these fliers is in the right place. But today I have no desire to pick one up and read it further. I do not need promotional packets. I am still caught in the theory that the best medical information is in the form of a kind old buzzard in yesterday's shirt who makes house calls and carries an *Antiques Road Show* kind of worn leather bag.

I have already gone to the Internet, pumped the nurses for additional information, pored over library self-help books. But, you see, I still carry false but comforting images of an era when those fellas took time to be totally present. Sat down, had some coffee, relayed necessary information tucked in between a doughnut bite and an inquiry about the new pet. His kindly presence gave meaning to a room where tears were allowed, where we had the full attention of the whole person sans billing clerks, waiting rooms, and piped-in music.

Can I make the transition to our impersonal paper-generated society?

UPKEEP

Grass grows whether you're sick or well, though gardening, fortunately, can be limited to window boxes. They were the first things we added to our quiet old picturesque farmhouse, and I guess they will be the last flourishing, exuberant gardens that we tend: vinca, bright petunias, fuchsia geraniums, minute drippings of deep blue nodding lobelia.

Outdoor upkeep has conditions. Bending over is nice with a helpful hand. Carrying heavy watering cans is possible if they're half full and if someone has been kind enough to connect that ancient old hose to the inconvenient spigot.

When we take in the sweeping view of our large lot, we realize that much has been freely given. We are thankful for all the colorful perennials in the fall, that border our yard and require nothing from us but appreciation: the vibrant sumac, the flowering shrubs, the wild daisies, the wisteria on the gazebo. And potted geraniums in summer and a basket of bought chrysanthemums in fall.

We now have time to look more up than down, absorb bright skies, and cheerful birds in flight and forget about trowels and drainage.

PAIN

The stupid sign on the cubicle wall says "are you in pain?" demanding that the patient gauge the severity according to ten degrees there on a charted pastel time line.

As I said, I think that's a stupid question.

Each of us—sick, well, or just bravely surviving—carries something unwanted, superfluous, or burdensome in mind, body, or spirit. Most of us find ways to bear it, dull it, or transcend it, from rampant busyness, or vodka martinis, to concentrated meditation. Or we take a pill, or play let's pretend or focus on completing a favorite project via mind control. Common degrees of pain? Probably. Ability to verbalize? If necessary. (We already know the difference between a blizzard, a squall, and a whiteout.)

Some of us were brought up to believe that good behavior and intelligent decisions guaranteed painless success. So we had to grow up in a hurry when we discovered that bearing discomfort could be a normal part of a person's day.

BEACH HOUSE

I think only God can organize the use of a family beach house. Jointly shared by a very large family, it is where wet bathing suits and sandy feet parade throughout, and youngsters can drop damp things without fear of reprimand.

We sign up early each year, David and I, to declare our preference for a certain week or two in July because there is great demand for the mammoth place for anniversaries, birthdays, weddings, church gatherings, and overnights, with dinner parties a colorful cross-stitch of family dynamics.

Of course, paying the bills and cleaning up divide the family sheep from the family goats! Because David and I live the closest—twenty minutes away—we often find ourselves replacing the screens or items that no longer work.

To some of the adult women, it is not a vacation. But watching the glee of grandchildren and the gaiety of guests absorbing the vast coastal view for the very first time always makes the commotion and preparation worthwhile.

Now I am thankful that this place with its many joyful faces will be able to nourish David during these difficult years ahead.

ROUTINES

What happened to August? To summertime? The two-week treatment sequence takes on a beat of its own.

Each day, cross off calendar date and count the remaining. Each day, check clock, check oxygen. Get dressed but ignore hair. Supply fast breakfast but no time to eat it myself. Head for door after counting pills. Slide into car seat. Gas up today?

An excessive wait for a tardy appointment means a stanza of multiple choices.

Shall I sleep in the car in the parking lot? Sit in the waiting room with soiled copies of *Ladies' Home Journal*? Join four pale men, slumped into their own locked-up eerie thoughts? Run to the nearest Shop 'n Save for David's favorite entrée? The return chorus means pick up the forgotten milk and the new prescription. Drop onto an unoccupied couch to doze off. Another unchosen day to be performed lovingly tomorrow.

AMOS THE CAT

My old cat from the SPCA just had seven teeth removed. This loving, affectionate tiger lap cat is now swaying and languidly collapsing as he slowly aims his fifteen-pound weight across the blue and black wool braided rug toward me. (Diseased gums had required immediate action.) My heart aches for his obvious discomfort, and I stroke his thick variegated fur as he settles uncertainly beside me on the big red couch.

I think he both hates me and wants me—the two-legged caregiver who dishes out his portions of Elegant Entrée and Mixed Grill, and also carts him off to the vet in the big green carrying case. Yet he now sprawls on the couch, snuggling close beside me, sleep erratic and drooly, dreams bringing on occasional twitches. Doped up, he idly glances my way, seeming to smile.

Maybe it's a relief not to be able to question, to think, to clearly reason about the whys and wherefores. To block out dentist's taking of vitals, the forced slumber, the approach of needles, the embarrassing leakage. But for those of us humans waiting and watching with our loved ones before and after the medical procedures, the cerebral ticktocking is hell, all concerned reflection ground down by possible complications and irreversible conditions subverting our patience.

NURSING

I am impressed by certain support staff at the cancer center. They consistently maintain a positive levity and clucks of concern to our moods and grumpiness. How do they do it? Rooms full of silent, suffering heroes, medicinal smells, and oceans of paperwork, yet they cheerfully decorate the place come Halloween with comical bats and before Christmas with evergreen trees boasting cheerful swags.

Historian Theodore Zeldin says there was once "little respect for those who took care of the physical needs of the sick," that this was a task normally left to widows, fallen women, and unemployed who were often "unpaid, given only shelter and food."

Today, nursing makes me wonder about the endless youngsters officiously tending computers and phones. Do they know they are *not* building close personal, caring relationship? Do they become immune to the sight of struggling spirits inside weakening bodies? When we hear that we are in dire need of nurses, is it because the real expression of care required in bedside nursing is too demanding or because their specialized skills are not appreciated?

We are all ministers to one another. When we do not wear black robes and quote scripture, we may need other visual reminders, such as acknowledging one another in casual friendliness and exhibiting patience when an emergency backs up the waiting room to standing room only.

Is nursing a special kind of calling?

CHRISTMAS I

How shall David and I observe Christmas? What dare we omit? What is essential to our inner needs, and what trinkets of consumerism can we discard? What is most meaningful to David?

We begin by deciding what we will not do, as in wrapping and mailing packages to faraway folks. The post office routine, usually shared, would be exhausting for me. Purchase a giant tree again? How beautiful the last one had been, filling the corner by the fireplace in our high-ceilinged farmhouse. Lapsing into a potent and very nostalgic moment, I recall how granddaughters Jayne, Kayley, and Leah happily trimmed it, the arrangement of balls and bells delightfully asymmetrical.

We choose a four-foot tabletop tree, but then we discover that most of our ornaments are gargantuan. I make a fast trip to town to hunt down a few miniature ones. The finished effect is fine, but it is definitely small.

I write a Christmas letter, the first in years, highlighting not children's antics and achievements but an update of the latest medical information.

Betty, David's sister, visits, and we start a cozy tradition of working a picture puzzle by the fireplace.

We travel to Hanover, where David's brother Malcolm and his wife annually host a festive family buffet and gift exchange.

We all hold in our hearts delicate old traditions via memory as we proceed into the uncharted waters of another year.

CAMARADERIE

"How do you spell 'oncology'?"

We're in the waiting room again.

We meet in the cancer center and immediately establish what people call "rapport," meaning easily shared frank and open revelation of a rotten medical condition. Another patient, jolly and round, hopes that his thirteen-year-old daughter (he sees her only on weekends) will get the message that bowel cancer and consequential spreading could be avoided if she doesn't follow in his footsteps, meaning, "Quit smoking, sweetheart." For myself, I am glad that my husband has at last completed the similar rotten schedule of daily treatments and is now looking forward to a period of possible remission. This stranger is actually writing thank you notes!!!

We continue our talk about the *real* in blunt honesty and reduced phrases, having already sifted out the trite stuff of life and connected with a common denominator. The stranger says "good luck" as he turns to the arrival of his updated condition.

We all have important stories to tell. But sometimes our stories go only to strangers or into the adoring eyes of our trusting canine or feline.

CHURCH

Sometimes attending church by myself is a good thing. I bow to habit, heartily sing old familiars, ingest fatherly exhortations from the pulpit, smile, and show vague signs of welcoming parishioners' concerns.

Other times the process of Sunday attendance destroys me. I sit in silence in our favorite spot and sneak out before the doxology. I do not want to talk with the synthetic do-gooders or answer endless questions about David's current condition.

What is the matter? Any reason I couldn't just hand out a chart or copies of the latest medical reports?

When David and I first married, I was constantly quizzed by David's friends about Louie. My husband had taken in this old friend who was down on his luck, allowing him to live in his home for a significant time. And I had always been tempted to say to those random requests, "When did *you* help Louis?" Their inquiries always seemed a mockery; what appeared sincere was really regimented taught civility.

Good manners can seem artificial, bereft of genuine feeling. Robotic behavior, like my 11 a.m. Sunday attendance, can be a weak substitute for the real thing. Are my responses perhaps on a par with theirs?

How do I deal appropriately with innocent inquiries and at the same time worship with open conviction, not just habit?

ADAPTATIONS

The ingenuity of folks inspires me.

Consider:

David keeps his plastic urinal incognito within a winebag atop his walker bicycle basket.

Helen gets into the shower, naked, to help her grandmother bathe.

Alison sits on the floor with her wig off so that her young nieces can touch her bare head.

Ann puts the noisy concentrator in the basement and runs the oxygen tube up the laundry shoot.

I keep a kitchen stepladder in our pickup truck so I can climb aboard in an emergency to fill David's small portable oxygen tank from the large liquid oxygen barrel kept there.

THE NOW

Comedian George Carlin says we have no "now." There are only sequels, reruns, remakes. My mother saved surprises for the future in the bottom drawers and labeled things from the past in cardboard boxes.

Why is it difficult to live in the moment?

If the past represents only regret, and the future only fear, why don't we make the most of "the now"? What is more important than this time together. Hearing gossip about a neighbor? Attending a cocktail party? Comparing the price of tuna at Shaw's and Market Basket? I don't think so. Yes, the "now" for the caregiver requires flexible planning, instant prioritizing, a lot of physical exertion. But this moment will never come again. If I go to bed imagining that this is our last night together, perhaps when it doesn't turn out to be so, the getting up can be joyfully received.

The "now" is becoming bejeweled with priceless value.

VISITORS

Occasionally I invite friends from away to join us for lunch. At home is best for get-togethers with David as he can simply excuse himself when necessary and go up to bed. I really like having guests. After traveling the distance I silently applaud their making the effort and have learned how to keep the process easy.

I make an apple or a blueberry pie, for which I have a decent reputation, and usually dash over to Weathervane to pick up some fresh lobster for a succulent salad or sandwiches. Then the four of us can sit around the old pine drop leaf table in the wainscoted dining room with the squeaky floorboards and the cheerful drapes I made. We can pretend for a little while. With Yale classmates Perry and Alison or Frank and Bonnie, it is easy. The conversation is usually mock carefree and lively.

Today it is to be Charlotte and Ian, Canterbury friends. After Ian's reference to his anniversary celebration, he gets an admonition from his Alzheimer's wife of a "Why didn't you tell me?" giving us a momentary excuse to diplomatically smile.

We all live in some kind of pretense, I say to myself. Unlike Brother Lawrence who happily served in the kitchen, I have momentary trouble practicing the presence of God as I collect the empty plates and wash the dishes.

YESTERDAYS I

I agree with the hero of self-reliance today who said "sickness is a cannibal" as I grab a recall or two from our past happiness.

I remember our first years in our renovated Canterbury cape surrounded by millennial stone walls, ancient rhubarb, wooded trails, vast fields for cross-country skiing, and a pond out back where David taught the young grandsons Ian and Steve to skate by pushing a clutched kitchen chair. It was a place where rural life meant such joyful proximity to animal antics: the dog's repeated tangle with porcupines, the owl who knocked himself out by misjudging a window, the giant turtle with shoreline-burrowing habits, the rumble of runaway horses streaking across our lawn. The sleepy town was aglow with a Shaker ambiance, and we labored at Saturday fairs in July, and sang/danced our hearts out in Gilbert and Sullivan productions.

Then there was my commute to the Boston area for my master's degree and at graduation the old rental on the Maine coast with our dog Cecil where each late afternoon meant lugging canvas chairs and a thermos of martinis to the sparkling white sands of Goose Rocks Beach.

We chose the casual and the occasional over endless comments such as "Why don't you travel more?"

Practical and psychic to the core, following our bliss became the saving for medical expenses.

RHYTHMS

My grandmother Clark in Bethel, Maine, believed in punctuality, on her terms. If you didn't show up for breakfast at seven, you didn't get any. Only her timepiece counted.

Life, of course, gives us all an inborn sense of rhythm. As children it was "the wheels on the bus go round and round" or babies rocking or bouncing to the beat of ragtime or Mother Goose. Then it was the sway of the waltz, the swing of the baseball pitch, the stamp of the foot to the beat of the band. From birth to death, movements have been provided that give us a universal sense of harmony. Likewise, most of us have established a comfortable individualized daily routine, whether it's rising early or staying up late.

My life as a caregiver skews up my own personal sense of rhythm. When caring for another, the time frames get set and the caregiver eventually learns to adapt and focus on providing comfort for the welfare of the patient. Well, I am slowly learning to adjust to the rhythms of David's needs only. The world of regular schedules or dependency on plans carefully laid sink away as other priorities sprout that required our immediate attention.

The hands of the Seth Thomas clock or the Longine watch do not compare to the adjustable switch to the hands of love.

PSYCHOLOGIST

She is trained to listen with a "third ear" to our woes. Because we don't want to burden our families with thoughts of desperation, we caregivers may seek out her safety net to get razor sharp awareness at an hourly rate. We are given permission to weep buckets or scream epithets. Yet she sits calmly, slowly forming short appropriate responses or questions, masking all her reactions to our mumbles.

Feeling safe behind closed doors and windows, we discover that we spasmodically know how to blurt out the unexpected, the rage, the fears, the unfairness of love stolen or cruelly wrenched from us. In the womb-like space with her there, no TV or traffic blots out or camouflages the hidden unbearable aching within us.

I stumble out of the sparse room with the framed diplomas and the potted plants that need watering. "Did I really say that?" I mutter to myself after having voiced an anxiety, yet I'm vaguely aware that relief was also part of the picture.

How much does she really care? Is she already thinking about that screwed-up next patient? Am I paranoid?

I float out actually breathing easier, at least for an hour or so.

ABBREVIATIONS

My husband shaves, if possible, before a hospital visit. He believes that if he is not neat and clean and medically smart, they will slap some sort of abbreviated sign on his bed that translates "Do not resuscitate."

DOA TFB CODE BLUE IMF

Think of all those acronyms in current usage. Impersonal? Yes. Time efficient? Maybe. But does relaying information in code make us better people? Where is this kind of language leading us?

I think sick folks and their families should design their own codes. Academia has its scholarly charts and medicine has its pharmaceutical lists.

Yes, let's make up our own. Let them figure it out!

I know what David's YLH always means.

DEATH I

I had never figured out what death meant aside from its devastating sense of void.

To add to the confusion, Christianity gives us a twofold view of heaven. It threatens some punishment and it offers relief. Now that death is hovering around again, what shall I do?

I was raised by Victorian parents who never took me to funerals and never talked about dying in front of me. But when my daughter Laurie's favorite elementary school teacher was killed in an auto crash, she begged me to take her to the funeral. I did. I saw firsthand how painful yet cathartic it could be, even though our going was unpopular with the other parents. Of course my husband at the time also knew how to take her in his arms and help her bear it.

I still seem stuck on the "why" of death.

I know only that I am not immune because of familiarity. It is not like piano practicing, as in the more you experience it, the easier it is.

Accumulation for me is destructive and hateful.

HOSPITALS

We've arrived again in Oz, at the hospital. Because of the distance to be traveled within the building, I help David into a waiting wheelchair and we roll into the footlights of our Broadway matinee.

Behind the scenes for us does not mean jaunty theater antics or a dramatically draped curtained stage. The props are not an exotic castle or garden greenery with lilting tunes, dwarfed choristers, or jolly actors with comical lion or tin man costumes.

The hospital today has a drab interior, an underground atmosphere, a crowded gift shop, a lengthy hallway with railings, color-coded drawers, labeled cabinets, wheeled carts, elevators, masked strangers, crews that mop—not photograph, and a highway of weary linoleum, not enchanting yellow brick.

Without red shoes, a barking Toto, or a high-pitched musical rhyming, the time for us here smacks of treeless and mechanical wellness, sterile technological systems, and polite mannequins going through the motions. But then a real voice magically broadcasts "Mr. Swenson?" I halt my foolish meandering, wake my nodding-off husband, and we roll onstage to appear before the latest remedial wizard.

REFRIGERATORS

My refrigerator reflects my present state: lettuce that shriveled too soon, a jelly gift dated 1994, cottage cheese with green "decorations," half a bottle of chocolate milk for a pick-me-up, something that used to be something else, four kinds of mayonnaise, and a tired tomato.

Caregivers know about takeout, pickup, and skipping meals altogether when we're too overwhelmed to plan, purchase, and prepare the kinds of foods we both can eat.

In truth, food is not a priority for those of us hanging in there. Appetites take a backseat to what's going on. We both eat smaller portions and thank God for those who lovingly drop off the home-made soup or the casserole with yummy melted cheese on top.

SICKNESS EXPRESSIONS

Doing poorly
Round the corner
Early demise
Not long for this world
Infirm
Sick as a dog
Under the weather
Looking green
Come down with
Laid up
Indisposed
In a bad way
Languishing
Pick up a bug
Holding his own

Evidently we think joking or slang phrasing will be enough so we can go back to our pretense of living. Is that avoidance? If we laugh about it, maybe it will go away?

DUMP

I make a dump run today. It was one of David's favorite Saturday jaunts, and as I rattle along in his old blue Dodge pickup, I wish he were the one doing it now. These excursions usually trigger idle thoughts, as in, what will be thrown away as time goes on? If diapers and tables are disposable now, will it someday be some of us?

New Englanders like to make these trips because they have a nose for spotting a bargain or exchanging exotic stuff. Like women who buy one anothers' junk at white elephant sales, men find delight trading discarded window frames, broken tools, and other basement castoffs.

Our dump staff are very helpful and maintain a pleasant repartee with residents amidst the mountains of bagged garbage, doorless refrigerators, metal scraps, building materials, and #5 bottles. So we exchange friendly greetings as I toss a bag here, a dissembled carton there, and even add an old framed print to the intriguing Swap Shop miscellany.

It is a fascinating place that is good for a little low-key chitchat and for political candidates to make a casual appearance.

Today, good-natured Bonnie and Ray ask for David. They know him as the nice man with the big dog who knew how to trade a lawn roller for a motorcycle. Not for himself, of course, but for his grandson Steven.

KEEPING UP

The social niceties of the BBC TV show *Keeping Up Appearances* seem trite to us native New Englanders who seldom worry about "proper" but think twice about a broken plow or a tasteless biscuit.

My brother, age eighty, complains he can no longer chop his eight chords of wood or plant his sizable vegetable garden. An independent artist who once skied in the famous 10th Mountain Division of World War II, he lives happily in rural Maine. But now his inquiries about winter rentals (his Thoreau-like existence can be rather chilly) bring responses of "no pets, no smoking, and no late night racket." But because his white cat, his violin, and his pipe are things he refuses to give up, he will just tough it out stoically because he's a real Yankee!

Then there's my clergy friend who says he can no longer keep up with all the changes in the church; and there's the widow who finds the endless increase in postage costs more than she can handle.

What does all this mean to people like me? When those who are relatively well are having difficulties mapping out their lives and keeping up with all the changes, what about keeping up when illness prevents normal involvement in common functions of everyday living?

CATALOGS

They sneak into the house with a new kind of product. I mean those color-coordinated consumer-oriented catalogs. Someone out there in the consumer world knows that tons of us need aids more realistic than trendy styles; we need textures based on warmth, not an see-through filmy. Models in these catalogs are not slinky thin, and merchandise does not include succulent fruit with holiday glamour. Instead, there are ugly shoes cushioned for comfort and childlike clocks with oversize numbers.

Yes, we need practical—gadgets for plucking dropped objects from the floor.

Yes, we need comfort and good fit—an elasticized waist and washable fabrics—but we also need the same intangible things as everyone else. There's just something sad about it all. And how did they know that David and I might now qualify for all those senioromics?

Is it my imagination that by providing the hushed about practical kinds of things, these entrepreneurs only appear to care about us, and are the shrewd ones making a significant financial profit?

MEDICAL HISTORY

From behind a desk I am handed a clipboard, pen, and sheaf of papers by a battery-operated girl with a sequence of nods. Yes, just fill out the forms. No, information about David's past is not on this computer. He, waiting patiently in the wheelchair, does not wish to do this again. In fact, he gives me a disgusted grunt. We have done this so many times.

I scan the same old list on the patient history questionnaire asking me to "check if you have the following medical conditions":

"Edema, renal failure, high blood pressure, sickle cell anemia. And questions "are you claustrophobic, are you allergic to shellfish, are you diabetic?" I could almost write up the form myself and wonder how they keep track of the endless paperwork.

Then it's the registration consent:

"I request treatment at the hospital and voluntarily consent to the rendering of such care, including diagnostic and surgical processes and medical treatment by authorized agents, physicians, and employees as may in their judgment be deemed necessary."

And of course, "I hereby authorize payment directly to . . ." Then there's the "Advance Directive Acknowledgment."

I guess David is officially sick when his completed paperwork is again accepted into their files.

PILLOWS

Why is it so hard to find the perfect pillow? There seems to be only unbendable foam; a loose sack of somebody's feathers; and a pillow too long to fit the standard case. David is poring over catalogs, seeking his favorite soft kind of punchable down.

I had just bought a gorgeous decorative pillow—silk embroidered with hundreds of tiny beads. Rust in color, it had called out to me there on the *T.J. Maxx* shelf and now sits on the couch in silent glitter and elegant design, a breath of singular beauty in a world of antiseptics, endless plastic refills, and mechanical breathing machines.

Pillows! The sleep shops give us sight of pristine unslept-in beds and smoothed-out bedding. The magazine ads give us pictures of glamorous, matching luxurious sheets and shams, coverlets, and ruffles. But have you ever seen a bedroom that looked like all those advertisements?

A bed does become central to sickness, a familiar place of comfort and rest. In spite of suggestions to the contrary, we continue to share the same one. Our bed is kept clean, but it is seldom picturesque like those ads.

History tells us that royalty once received callers while stretched out amidst lavish quilted bed linens. As David is now resting atop a premium goose down pillow I found for him, he can officially hold court, receive random visitors in true medieval fashion, though the hidden label on the mattress proudly reads Sealy Posturepedic.

IT'S A GOOD DAY IF

I've helped David take a shower.

I've thrown in a load of wash before breakfast.

I hear pleasure in David's voice because Elna or Mark has called.

The mail brings an outside connection unrelated to money.

Masterpiece Theatre promises the expectation of quality for the evening.

The cat Amos didn't throw up that new kind of urinary tract food for senior felines.

I climbed the stairs only twice, so muscle leg cramps will not keep me tossing all night.

GETTING SICK MYSELF

I get the flu, which becomes a rude awakening to us both.

Accustomed to good health and generally strong physical stamina, I had not planned for alternate caregiving. As a result we had a weekend that could only be called a Mack Sennett comedy of bleak survival!

I cough till my ribs ache. The cat Amos, impatient, traipses over us in bed, not liking his breakfasts late. David finds that heating up a can of Campbell's soup becomes a major challenge. He struggles to bring me the simplest of comforts. One day, coat over nightgown, I stagger outside to retrieve his newspaper. Dishes and garbage collect themselves.

How painful it was for David to realize how dependent he is. I need rest and temporary oblivion, but by Tuesday I am thankful just for standing stably upright. Knowing I can get better partly does the trick.

On Wednesday I pretend I feel great, suck in any sign of weakness, and click back into overdrive.

Sometimes we women just feel like trucks.

TRANQUILIZERS

I study claims, aka advertisements, about the benefits of medicinal drug relief to those of us sinking into unwanted depression. There is so much small print, so many names: Lorazepam, Temazapam, Paxil.

I am advised that a low dose and a gentle beginning started now will ease some of my agony ahead. You see, I know what is looming. The fact that my first husband also had cancer—a different kind— teaches me about the possibility of a long, frightening journey of gradual decline and hospitalization. So now I am reflecting on the updated medical system with all its advances supposed to relieve discomfort, but with its emphasis on prevention, not cure.

Uncertainty and curiosity about tranquilizers prevails. How do I put aside outdated attitudes of "just be stoic" or "don't be sick your-self" and intellectually consider how to be totally present and able to function in the care of my beloved.

My doctor is a kind woman, deeply concerned that I must go through such misery a second time, and she prescribes a modest temporary solution. And I compromise her solution by cutting the dosage in half.

HOCKEY

We watch TV hockey come winter. I am so glad to see David's happy absorption in a favorite sport. He was once both a fine player and a children's coach. His face reflects firsthand knowledge, memory, and experience. We get out class photos of team sports from the past, David posing with stick and puck, all eager and young and competitive in a lettered sweater and a funny haircut.

Sometimes these days he is taken to a UNH game by Jerry or cousin Tom. An elevator in the new Whittemore Arena makes this outing possible.

David does not focus on fancy equipment or yelling fans. His enjoyment ties back to fond afternoons on Turkey Pond in Concord dressed in brother Andy's secondhand skates and sweater. Years of intense living taught him what is really important in the playing—camaraderie and sportsmanlike behavior—with his adult counter-intelligence experience reaffirming that real living is done in plain clothes, a game is a game, and the recollected joy is in the simplicity of competing team friendships out in New Hampshire's brisk air.

SUNNY WINDOWS

We make the most of a window.

Fortunate to have big, high Victorian farmhouse types that let in light all day from one direction or another, we like to sit by, read by, eat by these openings, believing that all wide open places are capable of sending brilliance in.

We breakfast near the window where the bird feeder sways with fluttering activity.

We can bask in afternoon views of the river, or loll in a bedroom where, propped up, we feel the afternoon sunlight streaming in. Breathtaking sunsets fill up our cloistered, hungry souls with gladness. To easily see out is assurance that another world exists.

Is it any wonder that many cultures worship the sun? Is it a surprise that children adore window seats? Or adults covet the corner offices that open up great expanses of clear sparkling glass?

The terminal patient, the invalid—just like everyone else—wants to bask in, see, feel, and reverently touch the warmth and the brightness of that golden cream sauce that enriches the burdened life.

TAI CHI

What do you do for yourself is a question often thrown at me when I least expect it. I struggle to find an easy response.

Sometimes I remember to say "I'm studying Tai Chi. Seriously." (Not the watered-down lessons designed for elders.) That in turn brings a vague look of bewilderment.

If I clarify by adding "It's a wonderful mind/body/soul thing done barefoot and with no talking allowed," they sometimes show a bit of admiration. Then I get carried away and try a more dignified definition, and zero in on the centering, the focus, the satisfaction of "forms" repeatedly practiced, with the challenge to strive on and on and on to perfect the full body movements. But when I go too far and say that Tai Chi reduces stress or that it can be done alone in the middle of the night when sleep evades me, the description seems to defy their imagination.

I take group and private lessons, ignoring the cost because we both feel that the benefits are real. I actually heard David tell his friends that he could see a difference in me when I returned from the regimen of such focused classes.

I like the way the teacher always closes the twenty-four short form with the words "and returning to everlasting peace."

STAIR CHAIR

"You try it first."

Our excitement for the day is the installation of a stair chair. As we are fortunate to have a "straight shot" stairway in our old colonial farmhouse, it is just a case of my collecting technical information about price and availability. Purchased secondhand and guaranteed a buyback, we chose a model that is practical for us and fun for the grandchildren.

For the guest in denial about age, it means a hasty retreat and a "no thanks, not me."

For David it's a welcome relief to be able to rise to his bedroom, bath, and office, except for the accidental and noisy crushing demise of his favorite glasses that one day.

For me, things like laundry and suitcases get a ride in arms other than mine as I sing "Up, Up and Away in My Beautiful Balloon."

ANGER

I tried to vacuum up the shards of anger today. The specks of self-pity and clumps of anger must stay hidden. When he is so brave in the handling of disability and terminal illness, I cannot let go, let him see me like this. Luckily, he is sleeping soundly, upstairs.

The noise of the Miele helps to cover the feelings held prisoner so long within my tired psyche. Feelings of unfairness, someone dearly loved being snatched away, one's life put on hold, or rearranged, or attacked by predators.

The hum of the to-and-fro movement hides my excruciating anguish.

What did I do to deserve this? *Again?*

I push and pull the monster on wheels, yanking it around savagely, banging furniture, dragging the tank, hearing it greedily suck up the stray quilting pins and what is left from yesterday's living.

Others tell me of punching pillow techniques or talking to empty chairs, but they fail to convince me of the success of such methods.

A headstone from history roars into mind. "It was rumored his favorite word was damn!"

GRATEFULNESS

Today I feel grateful, cloaked in positives. Where does the change of mood come from? The weather? A good night's rest?

The simplest things feel pleasurable. A shared joke, a plain meal, reading our Sunday newspapers together (his the *Union Leader*, myself the *New York Times*) by the long bay windows in the living room casting the bright sun upon our panoramic and peaceful view of Oyster River.

I feel able to treasure each moment with the man I adore because these moments could be all we'll have, and they must last. Must, as the song says, stay "stored in a bottle."

"It doesn't matter, matter, matter, matter, matter," says the Gilbert and Sullivan musical ditty. And I will put together a simple meal of salad and soup on a tray and we will sit by the cozy glow of the old fireplace and pretend this is forever. Which it is.

No one can take my precious memories now being created. They can take my favorite blue blouse, my last year's tax returns, and my Hershey bar in the silverware drawer, but they cannot have these treasured moments in this homey space with my beloved.

FUNERALS

We attend a funeral today.

It is, of course, a physical struggle for David to attend, but I drive him to the door (all handicap parking spots are taken) as, determined to honor our church friend, he manages bravely with his folding chair cane. Dressed in a crisp white shirt and his only good suit, he believes staunchly that folks should not dress casually as they show their respect.

My thoughts are mainly with Paul's wife, Dot. I'm curious as to how others handle grief. Watching, I marvel at her ability to softly converse with endless acquaintances, and I recollect their unique late life marriage and their unabashed holding of hands—she five foot one, he six foot two.

For me, funerals have always meant showing up in clean clothes before a spiritual leader who must stand up there and soothe us as we're stumbling in terminal darkness. Like the blind being led to water, we need to drink assurance, and trust in the directions offered.

Discussion on the return trip centers on what we want or don't want for our own services. He wants a lot of references to his soul and does not like the current tendency toward informality—endless jumping up with recitals of anecdotes and pranks. I like to hear mentioned what was real about the deceased. Yet we agree it is a very sacred time, demanding appropriate worship and beautiful music that transcends the carefully vacuumed space of the moment.

DREAMS I

We pride ourselves on dealing well with one more day. Then the strange dreams dot our nightly slumber with both funny and terrorizing stuff. Last night it seems I screamed out, "They're killing him, one pill at a time."

That is somewhat easy for me to analyze as I spent time yesterday cleaning out our upstairs medicine cabinet, as well as evaluating the large assortment of pill bottles kept on the kitchen table in a handy basket.

He, in turn, cried out that the roof is falling in—also easy to analyze because his family has just decided to part with the well-used-jointly owned beach house.

Roofs falling in is an interesting metaphor that can apply to a surprising number of life events or circumstances. Where does the phrase come from? Why are we not more apt to say "falling down?" Is it because we are really dealing with inner things, things of the heart? Or is it about exteriors that are not important? A reminder that within each of us are issues we are afraid to discuss?

WAITING

I'm obsessed with the word "waiting." Others through time have already given the word considerable service. The famous stage play *Waiting for Godot* by Samuel Beckett, spoke to the issue; Simone Weil's *Waiting for God* spelled out her lifetime search for meaning, which she eventually found in service to the very poor.

We all once waited for boyfriends to call, cakes to rise, and small children to use the bathroom. A friend once said her teenage son ate two sandwiches while waiting for the toast to come up!

I, too, now do my share. I get tired of waiting in grocery lines and traffic lanes. I want to get things done so I can get on with my demanding real, daily life.

Today, I am impatiently waiting for the doctor to call back.

911

When the grocery tally came to nine dollars and eleven cents, the new young clerk said, "I hope you don't ever have to call that number!"

"I already have . . . three times," I calmly said.

"Why?"

"My husband has severe breathing difficulties."

"What's his name?"

"David."

"I'll pray for him."

My day renewed by astonishment.

NAPPING

David's napping is a signal that I can get the dishes done, the laundry collected, or more likely that, I, too, can retreat for a while by stretching out fully clothed and able to forget the recent sight at the hospital of a bald child or a legless man.

David and I both do free-form napping. Nine to five schedules have become obsolete. When his body is tired he lies down, be it 10 a.m., 2 p.m., or late afternoon when thoughts of an evening meal flicker and fade.

There are naps in the car, naps in the chair during the world news reporting, naps during boring conversation about sports figures' obscene salaries or the latest teen antics.

So when I came across the charming little book *The Art of Napping,* I laughed out loud!

According to the author, we live in a nappist society. There is synchronized napping, a napping style, and the family that naps together. There are even eccentric napping habits of famous people.

The next time I feel guilty before a snooze, I will remember the author's delightful enjoinder: "On the seventh day, God nappeth."

UNDERSTANDING

People do not understand about cancer.

They think that news about someone's recent diagnosis implies an imminent death. Or "that's too bad" is often followed by silent expectations of delivery to infinity, instant deportation to anomaly. Or friends with cancer often are written off to disappear to an assumed and immediate demise. Or is it fear of contagion?

It's not like that.

David and I are still here. Days become months, months stretch into years, hope is a fuzzy presence. In public, I mutter, "He's doing well, thank you" before exiting or changing the subject. Inside I'm thinking "don't pity us" or "you haven't the foggiest notion, and I'm too tired to explain."

Aggressive treatments and early detection are surprisingly successful sometimes.

A panel of doctors on TV recently said that people have a much higher rate of survival now than twenty years ago. Diversity of physical makeup, genes, and variable circumstances all contribute to the fate of each profile. There are remissions, meaning no cure but periods of no change either. There are plateaus of waiting, checkup dates fearfully noted, trips to seek second opinions. One dies, another passes the five-year mark and goes out to celebrate with a champagne dinner.

There are no guarantees.

We go on living while we wait for the Red Sox to win the pennant.

BAD DAY

I begin the day by dropping a plate on my foot. I am trying to do three things at once: unload the dishwasher, chat with David (propped at the kitchen table in front of his row of seven laid-out pills, and toast three slices of raisin bread before throwing in the laundry. This is just after I had again tripped over his fifty-foot oxygen cord, barely catching myself from a nasty fall against the counter. A choice word escapes from my sweet (ha) mouth, which causes Amos to wince, with ears back, and race for the cover of dining room darkness.

I sit down to evaluate the pain and peer at a blackening bruise on my right ankle bone. The possibility of being laid up for days in a quiet upstairs bedroom could be serious, but it would have definite merits.

The sight of the bruised ankle makes me think of my mother's protruding veins in her hands and legs as she aged. I had turned away, like most children, from that gnarled and aged look. Now, that vague repugnance, easily recalled, is joined by the fact that she had raised three children, and been on her feet in the inconvenient kitchen endless hours and without benefit of modern appliances. I remember only that I was never going to look like that! Now, here I am, hurriedly doing an appraisal of my old leg.

The discomfort fades as I realize I now know more about life than I once did.

BEACH II

I run away to my hideaway beach motel. My sister Mary Ella babysits.

It is November, and the off-season room opens directly onto the beach. I lock myself into a three-sided cocoon, pull the easy chair up to the sliding glass door, and inhale the expansive, welcoming ocean view in Maine.

The thunder of the surf instantly comforts me. "I am here," God's faithfulness murmurs as the repetitive tumbling onto the beach drums its eternal, roaring reminder.

A single gull appears and seems to adopt me. He sits on a railing in front of my unit, alone, expecting a donation. His squawking peers swoop overhead. He talks me into crumbs from yesterday's donut.

What is it about water? In rain, sun, or snow, its variable coloration is elegant, stable, vast, booming or peaceful. I bundle up, throw open the glass door, and join two happy dogs and a solitary walker. Hands in pockets, I silently glide along over limitless packed sand through unrestricted space.

The spirit of God descends upon my waters.

DOG SHOWS

The TV offers us a dog show series. The parade of furred specimens leashed to owners pacing the ring prompts me to playfully guess what a dog could be thinking.

"It seems I'm a winner." I pick up my gait and my tail on command, faking alert. The place is packed with crowded bleachers of anxious Homo sapiens who think my grooming is rather keen. I've been clipped, combed, shampooed, and jerked around before they run along beside me gasping for breath and praying that their body parts don't jostle too much.

They expect me to ignore other dogs also competing. How stupid! I obey only for the sake of those endless treats hastily produced from their fancy pockets. Just look at the heavyweight crackpot in Nikes and the snob in the sequined dress! The crowd is screaming. What a racket people make!

They do not know that I think the process is foolish, and only a desperate human would carry on this way in the eyes of so many of his mates.

Whoops, I need to piddle. Why *does* a mere blue ribbon make my owner so foolishly happy?

CAREGIVER TALK

Phone conversations with other caregivers are usually straight to the point, blatantly honest. We skip over niceties and zoom in to basics, blasting the day with relevance. It is a welcome exchange.

"I've just taken out insurance on myself," says Ann, who is worried about who will care for her hubby if anything happens to her.

"I've solved the dinner dilemma of decisions about preferred edible foods," says Peg, who writes out a week's possible menu, giving her dying husband a chance to pick and choose so that shopping and preparation time is minimal.

Women are marvels at adaptability and flexibility. We know that sharing what works for us may be helpful to another. We know that blowing off steam with someone who understands helps to relieve tensions.

Just the fact that someone is simply checking on us is uplifting. Advice is not the only purpose; it's the sound of a human voice, the sound of the short, "I was thinking of you today."

PAIRING

Male and female, Procter and Gamble, Sonny and Cher, Ben and Jerry. I am a victim of pair analogy. I try to rewrite the script: Woman with spouse at home. Woman with invisible husband. Widowed once and then again. Woman with cat, dog, or horse. Alien to grand marches, dancing partners, harmonious duets.

Having lost my first husband at an early age, I know all about being single in American culture. I'm talking about the exclusion from social life, the attitude of disdain. I'm talking about the man who says to the widow, "What you need is a good screw." Though I believe that much of this attitude is not intentional, we are part of a culture that paints reality as only youthful, jovially paired, and physically active.

Actual statistics about singles in our society are mind boggling. A significant percent of our population now lives alone. And while many make this choice deliberately, many others are victims of circumstances. Gilbert and Sullivan, there you are again!

HAIR LOSS

Memories of passionate lovemaking surface. Scorched visions of our honeymoon on that island, our leisurely weekends in our elegant renovated Canterbury house bedroom, tanned younger bodies lithe, whole, reaching, embracing, caressing, pulsating.

Now his dark, wavy hair I once ran my eager fingers through is gone. The handsome Omar Sharif look-alike is reduced to a semblance of the elder George C. Scott. "Maybe I'll get a new wig next," he jests after plucking clumps of long stray strands from our snowy white pillows. In truth, he simply chooses to wear a small, favorite hat, even to bed.

We laugh.

We say it isn't important. What's wrong with a turban, a visor, a ski cap, a scarf, or Dad's old fedora? Recollection of Holocaust victims changes the perspective. We become the lucky ones.

We remind ourselves that the folks in science are trying to help us, not kill us, doing their all-time best, often proceeding with fascinating new and successful treatments.

READING GROUP

I am privileged to still be part of a local reading group.

Morning coffee in Becky's living room means a short time away with good friends and good conversations about all manner of things. Even though the effort of dressing in presentable clothes can be trying, I want to attend and make the effort.

We are somewhat unconventional, which makes the group so inviting. Honest responses to "Did you like the book?" can make for some lively discussion. Besides, it's a university town and anything goes.

You see, without formal or staid leadership, we rely on the knowledge of all women present because we seem to represent such a rich and diverse background of interests and experience. The fact that one may not have read the book does not bring persecution, and often our comments drift off from plots and on to the latest political scandal. You could say we both educate ourselves and play, limiting ourselves in choice of subject only by what's available in paperback.

Sometimes it's folks like Ahab's wife or Shreve's ability to use a local setting or the heartbreak of the Hmong or the secrets of bees peppered with an occasional classic that inspires a hearty discussion.

The recent survival allegory of life on a raft with a tiger seems to speak volumes of truthfulness to me.

QUESTIONS

What is your Web site? Who do you have a crush on? What is your shoe size? Are you allergic to anything?

As we grow up, the questions do not have easy answers. We seem to have moved from direct and personal to devious and official or, for example, from cane to walker to wheelchair, all at a snail's pace. Before I self-destruct, I envision the typical progressions of inquiries about my life to include only vague questions that invite generalities, like, "Would you like to comment on . . . ?" Answers are no longer supposed to be yes, no, and maybe, and my anxiety seems to block the ability to spit out the expected details. The fact is ignored that we folks have advanced full circle from sandboxes to hayrides to mortgages to serious reflection of basics.

I prepare supper for us on a tray while MacNeil and his well-dressed guests ramble on about world disasters, talk to those on the home front, giving the illusion of company. They are lively, bright-eyed, and efficient interrogators, while David and I, veterans of lengthy life patrol, are just thankful for our ritual of easy and relevant questions and answers.

TANKS

Tanks rule our lives.

I am not talking about large army vehicles for military attack, or large white cylinders in the basement to guarantee that my bathwater will be hot. Nor am I referring to scuba diving equipment designed for underwater exploration, or giant underground storage tanks to hold quantities of gasoline for automotive consumption. Or water tanks held high on stilt-like structure and appear to come from outer space. Nor do I mean tank tops,—scant summer wear for sweet young girls.

I mean the small green kind. Containers that are life-giving to those with breathing problems. Or the large metallic ones for liquid oxygen, which we keep in our garage to be regularly filled so that we, in turn, can fill the portable tank on a strap that makes it possible for David to periodically leave the house.

David's ease in dealing with these tanks, concentrators, and inhalers carries over into thoughtful advice to others. He gets calls for help from friends, as the process for filling the small one can be tricky. Warnings about open flames and oxygen have upset me and others on seeing David with his cylinder in a room with smoking guests and decorative party candles.

I also keep an eye on the number of spare green cylinders kept here and there . . . for those of us who lose things—the miniature wrench to adjust the oxygen flow that can be tied onto the two-wheeled cart.

STEVE'S WEEKEND

Young grandson Steve, age seventeen, arrives in his black pickup truck purchased with his own savings. His energy, fast movements, and positive attitude about life are refreshing to us two struggling elders. We celebrate by lighting candles in the dining room, lugging out the "good" plates, and watching a hungry person eat.

For breakfast he eats half a coffee cake, and at 7 a.m. starts a full round of spring household jobs—adding screens on windows, sweeping the garage, raking, making trips to the dump and the hardware store, bringing up air conditioners from the basement, and mulching the rosebushes. He works steadily all day, stopping only for liquid refreshment. (How many Cokes can one person consume?) But after a hearty supper and a little TV, he goes to bed early, ready to follow the same busy routine the following day. Tomorrow it's dealing with the lawn furniture, and the bird feeders.

How lucky we are to have a young man who knows how to help, who asks if I know that Grandpa falls asleep in the car, a fellow who can zip up to us from the South Shore, through Boston traffic, without a complaint about all those rude drivers and those endless construction delays.

MILKSHAKES

I haul out the old blender and try mixing milkshakes. Drop in a few peach slices, a scoop of ice cream, a tablespoon of wheat germ, and two cups of milk (that's a wild guess.) The doctor has said to fatten him up with wholesome drinks. Biblical phrases about the fatted calf pass fleetingly into and out of my mind.

Milkshakes, once a costly snack to a teenager, is now a meal substitute for ailing patients. Canned commercial concoctions, like Ensure, flood the market, but it's the cold, thick mouthfuls made at home that bring back images of Haslam's Pharmacy in Melrose, Massachusetts, with memories of perching on high, wiggly stools before a marble counter top, and the tall metallic container soon to cough up a second foamy glass of peppermint frappe. We dealt out two dimes onto the shiny stone surface in exchange for the luxurious treat. I can taste it now.

But you cannot make a child eat, and you cannot force a husband who already drinks thirteen glasses of water a day, whose stomach is already distended by emphysema, who says his lungs are pushing down on his stomach, to gobble or drink every goodie provided.

EMERGENCY ROOM

Center stage, literally, is the discomfort of my sweetheart.

We are in the emergency room, curtained cubicle number 2, where wheeled stretchers on-the-ready crowd the corridors.

I look around, hastily, at our four walls of plastic hookups with shelves of unknowns packaged in their sterile wrappings, waiting. Pulled curtains that are supposed to veil privacy do not block out snatches of hushed conversations by staff and victim's next of kin. "Did you call Mother?" "How many did she take?" When I note color-coded instructions on the cubicle walls, I panic. Do the professionals here still need written instructions?

Frightened, I take a stand by the only chair while clumsily draped in David's jacket, my coat, his hat, my book, his newspaper, while clutching the hastily grabbed plastic sandwich bag containing his current meds.

The doctor on duty appears, discreetly solemn. Sparse words are exchanged as a glance in my direction brings an impersonal "We're going to do a few tests," which precedes his brisk exit from our imprisoned place.

We are left alone in the mechanized chamber, David hooked up to a blinking metal monitor that emits irregular bleeps.

What a relief when the nurse who bursts in happens to be a church friend!

QUILTING I

I linger over each quilt pattern because they are centering tools for me. Kind of a lectio divina. A book of 101 patterns promises hours of inspirational reflection though I have only snippets of time. Suggested sizes and colors invite grand speculation.

Quilting requires an active use of imagination. It involves brooding about, mulling over, sketching idly, pleasure in touching the fabric texture. Today I lose myself in envisioning a possible project. One large print, multicolor with two solids of sky blue and amber against a background of sea green and amethyst, or reverse the bold design so the background speaks as dark instead of light. Endless possibilities as swatches compared invite various color inventions.

Actually commencing an idea—deciding, measuring, cutting, and joining—is not possible at this time. Only silent involvement with patient deep-rooted life forces like time, beauty, and energy may breed eventual creations. In my experience prophets and quilters are in touch with the divine. Prophets—called to see what others do not spot among the injustices, the political turmoil; quilters—called to feel ecstasy in a stolen moment from the invading medical madness.

WATER

They've added a fish tank to the hospital waiting room. Miniature royal blue fishlets dart through clear waters made fairy-like with bright pink corals atop a base of glaring white gravel.

Who decided that waiting folk would enjoy this distraction? Why a tank of make-believe in this miserable place? Water, so often referenced these days only by threat of pollution, once signified only the Holy Spirit.

I look again at the tiny organisms effortlessly scooting back and forth and am reminded of dish soaking, foot washing, baptism by immersion, memories of beaches, playful dunking, and suddenly, is that a tiny new life venturing from behind the fake pastel coral-like tree form? Then more reflection, even wilder speculation.

"Look at me splash, mama," screams the little girl once again at the beach.

"Look at me die, daughter," says the silent old woman who needs a ritual of anointing as she departs a culture that merely blinks at her exhaustion.

WEDNESDAY

Wednesday is David's day out. Old friends who had also retired to the coast decide to regularly get together for lunch. They take turns picking up David—Dick, Tom, Buzz, Jerry, Ben, Charlie, Bert. Wives are supposed to be welcome but seldom join the trek to Ron's Clam Box or Joyce's Kitchen. The men do not choose linen/crystal types of places. They prefer informal where the potatoes are real and the pies are homemade.

When I asked later what conversation had transpired or what he had learned, his answers were fuzzy. I think the men relive some of their happy childhood escapades from Concord days, talk about a few waterfront issues like Tom's sleek new sailboat, and bet on UNH's chances of a hockey championship.

I love to think of their long-standing allegiance to one another, rare in these days of busy commitments. Their addictions to foodstuffs may seem limited: Tom needs his gravy, Dick his French fries, Charlie his blueberry pie. But their appetite for genuine, faithful friendship overflows their accumulated years.

READING IN BED

Over the years we have found great pleasure in bedtime reading. David enjoys professional and political magazines; I like various mystery writers. He prefers factual knowledge; I like some fantasy. I often scan; he ingests every word of every page in a book or local newspaper.

We read an occasional book review to each other, marveling at our mate's opposing viewpoints; sometimes this prompts exploring further evidence. Sometime we find avoidance is best.

Last week I bought him a book with true stories about our geographic areas he knows so well. Next it will be a Chinese auto-biography by Da Chen, an enchanting speaker heard on *Book TV* (David had done business in China.) These books will be followed by *The Professor and the Madman* and *The Hungry Ocean,* again about a New England subject. What we are enjoying together this week is the old classic *Arundel,* by Kenneth Roberts, a well-written look at hardy settlers of Maine who trudged north to Quebec during the American Revolution.

We are both surprised by a richness experienced from certain excerpts not personally chosen but entered into for the sake of the other, and I am saddened that his advancing hearing loss is beginning to erase this precious time of sharing.

STEEPLE

Our church steeple is in the parking lot. After years of benign neglect, and before space renovation and new construction, the tilting picturesque New England spire on our historic place of worship must be rebuilt. It's almost like a diagnosis of terminal illness.

The historic building, ravaged by time and moisture, is examined not on a high metal table but by a bustling batch of engineers, because it houses one of the oldest congregations in New England (1633), which is now in its fourth location in a prime downtown Dover location. The church membership declared that the mammoth clock and crowing rooster weathervane must somehow continue to be symbols to future generations. (I agreed to serve two years on the planning committee.)

The estimates on necessary renovation are staggering, but it must be handled by the best of professionals. Chaired by a friend and capable university professor, Nancy Kinner, the committee moves into action. Soon crowds are watching a giant crane and the assembling of great yellow scaffolding. For me, it seems to exemplify what medical care is about. Removal, renovation, and restructure—in faith, for the sake of a healthy new framework of hope for better tomorrows. In less privacy, of course.

THANKSGIVING

I am momentarily distracted as I note that red and green knick-knacks, not pumpkin masks, now clog the novelty stores. It is only November 3rd.

"Do I need red candles this year? Should I pick up some small gift exchange yet?" Then I pull myself together and get real.

Fall once meant making clever costumes for three children, then in November traveling to Goss Avenue to sit down for turkey in Mother's cramped dining room, with non-lumpy cranberry sauce served in her delicate pink glass compote. Later, Christmas meant jolly carols in stores guarded by bundled up Salvation Army ringers, and in adulthood candlelight services in St. Paul's Church, Concord, come midnight.

So Thanksgiving is again on the horizon, and I envision the grown children and their offspring happily gathered around, after making five pies and mashing ten pounds of potatoes. I know how worthwhile it all really will be, with a few changes.

Rick, my son-in-law, will carve the bird. Carolyn and Kayley will set the long pine drop leaf table with Indian corn, heirloom candle-sticks, and Leah's placecards. Everyone will help in the cleaning up as well as the eating, and David will delight in viewing the jolly turmoil before climbing regretfully aboard the stair chair to his second-floor haven of rest.

URINATING

We carry urinals in all car trips, long or short, so the sight of those plastic containers no longer embarrasses me. But it has shocked a relative or two who ran to remove youngsters from being entertained by the antics of an aging uncle.

My parents once made roadside stops when traveling in their 1940s Oldsmobile from Massachusetts to Maine. Everyone did. Rural back roads provided easy unobtrusive trees and bushes. Now, stuck on treeless highways and byways with only wire fences or metal railings, we make concerns regarding bathroom facilities a major priority.

How many architects now design homes and public buildings with specific convenience in mind? How many planners take into consideration what handicapped travelers often need easy accessibility?

In the meantime, David and I have been known to hurriedly veer off to a handy McDonald's or a rare roadside park while the car behind is probably ranting about those old folks who don't know how to drive.

ENVY

Does she pay her own rent? I am watching a woman who seems to be in charge of herself, poised, neatly put together in that stylish Liz Claiborne outfit. I stare and speculate. She certainly walks like she likes herself.

Who is she? Is her husband still at the office? Out of town? Mowing the lawn?

Deceased? Sleeping with her cousin?

Does she live in a grand house or an apartment on Market Street with a balcony view of the Piscataqua? Does she drink orange juice straight from the carton when she thinks no one is looking? Arrive at meetings early or late? Ever see her mother's face in the mirror? Sleep in curlers?

Or maybe she's single doing errands just for herself. Maybe the grand children's sweet faces are hanging there in the hall, posed and toothy, where she can greet them as she passes in and out.

If she is capable on the short-term care and feeding of child and husband, how will she act if someone in the family develops a lengthy illness? Will she, too, ever wear masks to disguise her reality?

I glance at my watch and hurry off to the filling station, grumbling, "Am I going to spend my whole darn life trying to figure things out?"

BACKWOODS

Most folks think of New Hampshire as a backwoods place where tourists dress up in L.L. Bean gear, do a little hiking, and ogle the natives. Where there's no sales tax but there's liable to be a big ugly moose ambling around. Actually, we're a bit more than that.

First, in New England we are good at naming things. Label bread under When Pigs Fly or name a store The Cracker Barrel or call a brewery Smuttynose. Second, we like certain basics, as in dry firewood and front porches bigger than a bread box. Third, we know how to make the most of a barn. We fill them with Flexible Flyers, rotting harnesses, wooden boats. Or we renovate the beasts into attractive but pricey living space. Of course, a few picturesquely seep onto calendars or quietly rot into our notoriously rocky ground.

There are a few things we don't know. Like, why do Dixville Notch folk get to vote first? Or why does downtown Durham have such a lousy traffic pattern? Or when did Dartmouth begin allowing girls?

What we do know is how to help out one another. That's our very best quality. But we'll always have prize words like "gundalow" to quiz the lurking tourist.

NOT A BILL

Did you ever receive an apparent demand for money during a "tight" period? In an envelope boasting a certain return address that made your heart go bumpity bump before you opened it? Though stated in heavy black Roman caps that THIS IS NOT A BILL, and while the document is clear and bold in its summary of expenses, your eyes race down the scary column and clamp onto the grisly numeric total of $10,040. When you get your breath and finally allow your attention to wander farther down the page, you locate the tiny print on the 8 by 10 poor-quality multiple-copied letter and eventually get the message that this humongous sum was already paid by Medicare last month.

David's response?

"Good grief," he exclaims. "I'm not worth that kind of money!"

At least his reply brings something to laugh about.

DREAMS II

I dream I am cleaning out a barn. It is filled not with manure and damaged goods but an amazing assortment of stuff, including varied fabrics in open cartons. In the dream I am rummaging through the mess, always surprised at the forgotten and the familiar. Things that had never been taken out after the last move. I was overwhelmed with a strange urge to lift out and display the hidden artsy things.

The barn in the dream is not a dark place. It is full of large openings and high windows and has plenty of brilliant light. Some people seem to drop by as I try to proceed with my very satisfying effort to sort and carry; others are intensely interested in my old treasures, bending over, peering, handling.

I have always been attracted to barns. But it is the quality of light in the dream that fascinates me most. It is almost heavenly in its welcome. After a lifetime of certain unresolved conflicts, can it be suggesting that the future could be brighter on Earth for me if I envisioned it positively instead of being dominated by feelings of pessimism and fear?

ANNIVERSARY

Amidst the demands of hospital visits and dump runs, I almost forget it.

But it promises a romantic day away with dinner out.

As I often do the driving now, I take David for a mid-day ride up the Maine coast. We both have a yearning to view the oceanfront; my wedding ring is a wide custom-made gold band of waves crashing, designed by Mark Knipe, a Concord goldsmith.

The York Beach area is a vast, wide open panorama, a welcome vista from inside our heated van. My job is to find a place with easy access for him, meaning no stairs, no gargantuan parking lots and no inconvenient bathrooms.

I find the perfect place with an enchanting menu. The new little restaurant, Safina's, is complete with recorded top-notch Dixieland music and plenty of privacy. I sip "our" token martini and look with adoration at my bald beloved smiling at me under my turquoise-colored fleece hat, his oxygen tubes dangling. Idyllic moments of pure joy, keen awareness of all we have had together.

We talk about the miraculous life we have had for eighteen years, assured that God must have been part of the plan, of our meeting, our marriage.

As we look into each other's eyes and experience our mysterious melding together, we let time stand still once again.

To love another person is to see the face of God.

MARY/MARTHA SYNDROME

Caregiving always makes me think of the famous biblical story about who was the best of two women—the one in the kitchen (Martha) or the woman sitting at Jesus' feet (Mary). I've decided that on a good day I can do both jobs—toss pots and pans around the kitchen in preparation for the hospitable role, and also sit quietly and absorb elusive facts and knowledge about faith.

Of course scholars have debated this dilemma ad nauseum, using it as a sounding board for sermons, with the cook in the kitchen usually getting short shift. Now in my real life, Martha's role has moved up a notch.

I am fortunate to have had three good friends named Mary, each a major part of a different chapter in my life—my college roommate, my neighbor from Lynnfield days, and my first friend made here in Durham. In childhood, my favorite Mary was Mary Poppins, who managed to toot in and out, up and down, touching others' lives just enough to change them.

Thank God for Miriam Winters. This scholar reminds us that both Mary and Martha images are neither attractive nor fair. Frenetic/withdrawn? Workaholic or insensitive to stress? Identity problems can go on and on. Doing our job means choosing our jobs.

FRUSTRATIONS

David cannot tolerate being unable to reach a doctor directly by phone. A Harvard Business School grad, he wants efficiency in all business transactions. So he faxes short inquiries, simple questions, and God knows what else. When he learns that his messages often sit for days in an unread slush pile before they are ever acknowledged, he gets furious.

On the next visit his doctor patiently describes how busy his staff is, and refers to a new technical updated system that will soon be installed to make it easier for us all.

Well, we don't understand their setups, old or new. When medical care costs so much, why should we have to understand the latest hardware? Why not a personal connection? What the heck are we paying for?

Words about waiting for results of medical tests drive him crazy, too.

DRIVING TO DOVER

I back the car out of the garage, shift into first, glide down our long asphalt driveway onto Route 4, take a fast right into busy traffic, and proceed one mile to the turnoff to Route 108, and head north.

Driving to Dover has become tedious. While I tire of these repetitious trips to the hospital appointments, I know I have chosen to accompany David so I can offer support on as many levels as possible. It's just the sameness of the panorama that gets to me—the same trailer park, the same delays behind the school busses, the red brick of the Woodman Institute, the Burger King with its Whopper aroma. If I vary the route slightly, I get to see the same broken fence near the Silver Street intersection.

Then there is the sameness of cemeteries, the Photosmith storefront whose owner is a chemotherapy compatriot, the same car wash. At this last, if Cecil is with us, we get to see in our dog's eyes the same kind of situational anxiety that sudden gushes of cascading water can cause.

We slow down in the ancient looping one-way traffic pattern, bump over the railroad track that crosses Main street, pass the drugstore that gobbles our prescription money like a hungry alligator, and finally arrive at the medical destination.

How do families repeatedly fit in this daily trek if their nine-to-five job is on the line?

STRONG

Over the years I have been called a strong woman. It is usually said with disdain, an implication of wrongdoing, an apparent preference to see me falling apart!

I review what has made me what I am today, both weak and strong. Parental influences—Pennsylvania mother, Mainiac father, and a pious upbringing. Being the youngest, being a Depression child, having an artistic temperament, and having a hard-won late education. Death of an infant son and first husband. Raw clergy family life in the 1950s and 1960s. A sweeping New England heritage that swaddled me in the practical and the sensible.

Well, I believe that all women can rise to the trying occasion, be it personal failure or a family crisis. If we are strong, it may be because we often have no choice!

Poet Marge Piercy says it well: "A strong woman is a mass of scar tissue."

HOT WEATHER

It is a sizzling ninety-eight degrees in early July. Folks call to see how David is coping. We tell them the upstairs air conditioner and home computer have crashed, but other than that we are fine. We do not say what a camera could tell them as we slowly move from room to room in loose-fitting, seedy, well-worn summer apparel. We guzzle down Paul Newman's fancy lemonade in desperation.

When I tell David I watered the mailboxes and picked the mail from the window box, we have a good laugh. Heat and old age produce strange dialogue.

We slow down our pace, and turn up the downstairs air conditioner.

We feel cool but claustrophobic. As we idly fume about confinement and forced inactivity, settling into our comfortable chairs, our conversation turns to how lucky we are, and we voice concern for the many who do not have a cool corner to fan hot tempers and feel relief.

Medical condition or not, it is just that we are not ready to become homebound. We do not remember deciding to become old and helpless.

CONFERENCE

I attend a one-day conference entitled "Caring, Spirituality, Healing" offered by a group of pastoral counselors and a cancer association. Four big names in therapy present stimulating viewpoints and discoveries. Their voices lift my spirits with their personalized sharing of facts/stories in which compassion seemed to be ruling their busy medical-centered day.

I tell friends that my purpose is to gather information for our benefit. What I gain is learning that many others with illness in the family are disconcerted by a profit-motivated medical system. Six and a half minutes is supposed to be allotted the average patient! The conference validates our feelings and experience.

It is good to know that there are professionals out there who really care about their patients, that listening is important, that biological fixes may not always be best, and that it's possible to provide the kind of relationships that heal the entire person: mind, body, and soul. It is also a relief to know that many in high places are aware that modern-day medical students must learn more about the lesser known interpersonal skills that can contribute to healing and wellness.

ECCENTRICITY

I like our license plate that says "Live Free or Die." A lot of people don't like it, and we get a lot of flack about it.

The truth is, we New Englanders have always liked the unconventional. Liked it when actress Jane Fonda in the movie *Julia* threw her typewriter out the window. Liked it when Shirley MacLaine wildly ranted at the nurse when her daughter, played by Debra Winger, was dying.

So who determines who is eccentric? With illness now part of living, David and I could adopt peculiar ways. Certain accepted norms and behavior may need to be dropped or buried. David is cold today though it is seventy-five degrees outside. He is wearing two old sweaters, a scarf I made for him, an ancient ski cap, knitted wool socks and heavy slip-on moccasins. The UNH teen who just walked past is in shorts, a T-shirt that says something political, and bare feet in plastic flip flops. Same day. Same town.

Our ability to adapt to climates and changing medical conditions is top-notch. Just watch out for what may be our own special unconventional behavior. For starters, in fear of germs, David doesn't want you to shake his hand. We certainly don't live by dress codes and little logos. We care less about what people think.

Besides, there is only one big label that matters. According to Rumi, "don't cover yourself with any garment but love."

THE RIVER

My friend and neighbor Harriet invites me to swim with her. Her property nearby borders the Oyster River with its saltwater inlet of refreshing current and its expanse of sky, occasional bird, and winding shoreline. I settle David down for his nap, then rush to grab a towel and rummage for a decent swimsuit for my old body.

The boat dock is long and hot under my bare feet. It seems like a century since I have walked in the open, barely clad. But I'm eager to test dip and sink down into the cooling depths. Can I still do it?

I back down the ladder, letting out a wolf-like howl of enjoyment. Has anything ever felt so good? It feels the same as when I was a teenager visiting my grandparents in Bethel, Maine, and I jumped into Songo Pond. It has been so long.

The miracle is that I can still stroke, breathe, kick, moving my body effortlessly forward. I roll over like a pampered seal, amazed, easing away any remaining anxiety about capability.

We talk in the water a bit before another foray to the next dock. The camaraderie of shared exercise lifts me to another sphere. Once an outdoor enthusiast, I realize that maybe, just maybe, my life may not be over, too.

The short drive home in a wet bathing suit is done in a state of euphoria.

TIME FRAMES

We are always late.

I try various strategies to get us to places on time: Tell him the appointment is 2:00 instead of 2:30 (it's not easy to lie considering my pious heritage); plan alternative outings when the first has gone by (it's hard for him to not rush freely as he pleases.)

I know he struggles just to get around. Every decision to move from one room to another room requires what feels like endless blocks of time. Every trip to the hospital means slowly getting in and out of the car, stopping frequently, allowing plenty of time to what he calls "recover" before another movement that requires effort to proceed to the next destination.

I get impatient with all the waiting around, but his lack of complaint keeps me mutely humble. So I learn to stop to also take a deep breath and to chitchat with him about whether the raccoon is still in our tree or why the bluebirds didn't return to eat the special grub worms we had carefully laid out.

SOUNDS

When out of range of noisy medical machines, like compressors, used by our loved ones, we enjoy any relief of silence, and return bolstered by the fact that if they can bear it, so can we. What has been called the least acknowledged of our senses now has become primary to me.

How much do we depend on sound? It seems to communicate warnings, pleasures, facts, or pressure. The cat Amos hears his tiny dish moved and dashes to investigate. When Carolyn visits, David asks for a song. An accomplished soprano, her voice expands his isolated space.

They say we grow accustomed to white noise, that it's all around us wherever we are—in traffic, on the subway, in a plane or the office. Lakeside lapping and children's laughter are rejuvenating, while dissonant department store music and family squabbles are disturbing.

When the noises stop, who will I be?

NUMBERS

This week or next? I must pay more attention.

Everything is numbered these days—rooms, phases, number of treatments, wins and losses, doses per day, TV channels, parking areas, seating arrangements, dental checkups. Then there are third Wednesdays, second Fridays, three-month referrals, and regular refills—if you can remember the prescription number and which pharmacy's phone is on the label.

My brain is becoming a network of forgotten figures. Lists and pocket calendars are supposed to be helpful reminders, so I begin carrying small notebooks with spaces for such essentials.

I realize that my once-handsome hero can no longer handle details. Yesterday's dosage or the morning phone call about a changed meeting date is easily forgotten. So I buy more notebooks, make out columns of dates and times and dosages, and pledge to be an accurate record keeper. But I know I am a right-brainer who functions with and trusts the spontaneous, and now I am called to pay attention to all these numbers.

God, help me.

SURVIVIOR DAY

We go to Cancer-Survivor Day in Dover. It is the annual barbecue sponsored by the hospital. I did not know what to expect, but David anticipates seeing those he had met through the rehab sessions there.

It turns out to be a balloon-blowing, live music, festive kind of occasion with hundreds of patients and their families partaking of grilled hamburgers, hot dogs, and mayhem. It's held outdoors at a spacious health club, where children splash in the pool and adults of all shapes, sizes and condition sprawl relaxed in folding chairs.

The hospital staff members, in cheerful yellow T-shirts, greet our familiar faces, and all attendees, ever hopeful, drop raffle tickets into temptingly described gift bags.

We all take turns absorbing sunshine, blue skies, and a temporary feeling of victory. "I made it" and "I'm actually still here" are heard as smiles communicate happy feelings.

"I think you won something, dear," David whispers as we prepare to leave.

"Me? Never!" I retort, laughing at the mere thought of winning.

But there on the giant board is my name. I win a $350 certificate to the Cliff House, an elegant beach resort on the rocky Ogunquit, Maine, coastline.

Praise God! A mini vacation to anticipate!

REMINDER

I'm feeling inadequate today.

By sheer chance I come across a startling reminder of my identity. On sorting some old desk files, I find a printed quote from Ecunet, the ecumenical computer network. The article creatively lists biblical characters and why they had seemed unsuitable candidates for their so-called leadership role. Moses stuttered, David had unacceptable moral character, Amos was a rural hick, Peter had a bad temper, Hosea's family life was a mess, John dressed like a hippie, and Jeremiah was too emotional.

I guess we can all forget that our qualifications for the job of loving and caring is often overlooked or defined by human terms. God's choices for us to serve in whatever is needed may not be our choice, but our job is simply to trust and follow. Special training may not be on our resume.

Today I will concentrate on feeling chosen.

DISCOURAGEMENT

We return to the old house after a treatment.

David slowly makes his way from the two-car garage through the mudroom to the kitchen, through the dining room to the front hall to the stair chair. We stop to discuss whether he's warm enough to take off his coat; should he be doing a nebulizer treatment before going upstairs; can he make it to the upstairs bathroom or should we use the urinal first. Note the use of 'we'.

I again silently reflect that it is all too much. Years of getting around for both of us is exhausting, and each immediate decision turns monumental. The downstairs half bath feels like it's a mile from everywhere. The closet is too far from the bathroom. The washing machine is too far from the bedroom. Why did we ever buy this house? Someone should tell the yuppies that owning a five-bedroom monster will eventually be a hardship.

I calmly switch his oxygen from the downstairs concentrator to the tube hooked by the stairs as I note that the six-foot-high windows in the dining room are in desperate need of a scrubbing.

Together, we vote for the upstairs destination but are forced to change, mid-stair, when the call to a bathroom becomes crucial.

WHAT MAINSTREAM?

I have been out of the mainstream so long that the world feels like a stranger.

The clerk in the store wears four earrings. Why?

The dairy section at the grocery store has been moved. Where is it?

The road on Route 4 near my house is being tarred. Why didn't someone warn me of the delay?

As I throw together another fattening dessert, I admit that flexibility must be mine if I am to live in this ever-changing world of extended life spans, chronic conditions, community changes. But when the *New York Times* tries to tell me about new boot styles, nouvelle cuisine and vacation trends, I tune it out.

David and I ignore the not fitting in.

We bask in what has been ours, together, so warm, so familiar. We treasure what we have shared: our similarities, the joys, the certain old-fashioned viewpoints, and then just let the strange new stuff roll by, off and away. Gilbert again?

AFTERNOON RIDE

The afternoon is ours.

We take a ride, the comforts of home riding with us. Though it is raining, we are cozy, cocooned in our merry Oldsmobile with the necessities of our current lives: folding cane, two umbrellas, an extra tank of O, sunglasses . . . just in case, an official auto handicap tag, a bottle of NH tokens, warm sweaters, binoculars, a urinal, bottles of water.

Then we decide, mid afternoon, to eat lunch with a view of the breakwater, gulls, marsh, and skyline. The fact that the deck at Saunders is closed is irrelevant. The restaurant, with its ship models and giant lobster tank, overlooks Rye's small harbor of sailboats, gently rocking. Like us, going nowhere.

What started out to be an errand day becomes a jewel of great price.

"I just like to be with you," David says to me in a golden moment.

ROLLER COASTER LIVING

There are bad days and good ones. There are weeks of relief and hopefulness, bouts of nausea, and weeks of just plain fear. Having grown up in Massachusetts not too far from Revere Beach's famous playground, memories of swirling Ferris wheels, slamming auto cars, and turning green on downhill rides can easily be recollected.

While we tend to believe what doctors tell us, we forget to note what they are not saying. Surprises can slam into us, even after a positive diagnosis. "Let's take another X-ray" is said as we wonder if the cancer is in remission or spreading to another location? "This treatment should give you another year."

"That treatment is only preventative."

"This treatment is highly recommended."

When "You're our poster boy" is finally tossed our way, our shared glance of disgust cables a silent "What ride will be offered next?"

But we retaliate. We take our own kind of ride, as I've already described.

It's an up and down world, and who knows what ride tomorrow will bring.

QUILTING II

Today I have a 50 percent off coupon for Jo-Ann's. It soothes me to take a short bypass to a fabric store when I am out grabbing the mish-mash of groceries. Walking the aisles where the hundreds of bolts of fabric for quilt making are displayed relaxes my senses.

The wide rainbow of orderly and smooth-to-the-touch fabrics are like friends to me. I randomly pull out a deep blue one—a beauty. I wonder what I have at home that would go with it? And justify my interest with isn't that the shade of green that is so difficult to find?

I have concluded that there are certain quilt patterns for our life stages. For me, now, it is the Cathedral Window pattern. Done by hand in small increments, and by folding small squares into sparks of bright colors, the finished quilt conveys the illusion of a large church window. It is a pattern to quietly work on when David is sleeping.

A quick glance at the store clock tells me its time to get back.

HIS ENDURANCE

Most of us connect the word survivor with a television program. The rest of us use it in reference to loved ones who—daily, weekly, yearly—practice a kind of courageous attitude that defies description.

"David, honey, how do you do it?"

As I watch David's patient endurance through endless treatments, I marvel at his inner fortitude and steady grit. Never a complaint, never a suggestion of giving up. Yet today he tells me to put him in a home.

I know what he really means.

He's personally disgusted that he cannot do more for himself, and feels he is a burden to me. He never wants to impose, always tries to do things for himself. Right now he does not like the recent development of needing help in dressing.

I reassure him that he's staying with me. To myself I say I want him to die with dignity at home because of the proximity of his loved ones, and because hospitals are increasingly seen as places of impersonal mechanical care. I recognize though that eventually professional help may be needed at home.

DINING ALONE

Stopping at a coastal hotel dining room for dinner causes the memories to flood back to the reality of what it will again be like to be a widow.

When my first husband died of cancer, I was 41. Eating in public places by myself was torture. Sometimes I took a book. Sometimes I just didn't eat out because single women are usually seated behind a pole or in a corner windowless or by the swinging door to the kitchen where the seething tempest of the back room clatter resonates.

Today, eating alone and easily remembering that kind of accommodation, I discover to my surprise that I have developed a new attitude. Am I more secure in my sense of self worth as a single human being? I know I have just as much right to be here as two yuppies and a noisy youngster in purple sweatpants! While a few bored glances do come my way, I seem to have moved beyond public expectation to some sort of surprising transformation. A little wisdom with age?

I daydream into a quilting intent to try my hand at creating those clever Prairie Point edges for my next quilt. Then I mull over the fact that my friend Ethel once said that she had discovered she actually liked her own company!

I'm hungry, I say to myself, and I know how to gobble down hearty fish chowder and a spectacular view just like everyone else.

RADIOLOGY

Some of these hospital spaces are a portrait of minimalism. How does the staff stand the sterile atmosphere? The plain floor tile, square biohazard floor containers, little steel boxes of cotton balls, the warren of cubby-holes. Even the stools and office size chairs seem to have been designed for metallic robots.

Then again, there are the changes.

Take the gizmo in the new radiology waiting room. Handheld, it is a cold mechanical object that lights up and vibrates to alert patients waiting their turn. It sufficiently jars you out of your reverie about last night's leftovers, tomorrow's women's meeting, and today keeping an eye on your mate's feet being safely placed in the wheelchair. While listening to an overdose of background music and scanning a dated issue of *Popular Mechanics*, you are also supposed to be alert to the behavior change of this black metallic creature!

How many new gizmos like this are there for the benefit of the patient?

Actually, it promotes a little conversation with the other victims.

AUTUMN

The brilliance of fall in New England beckons us outside with an excuse for short rides along the Maine coast to York, Ogunquit and Wells. I throw a few snacks, and two bottles of water into the car and we're off. David may doze, but so what?

The official fall foliage weekend has brought record-breaking crowds (350,000 as reported) up Interstates 93 and 95 to our glorious New Hampshire, and we find ourselves again saying how lucky we are to be able to live year round in a region that: boasts picturesque mountains, rivers and coastline bathed in colorful brilliance; and that provides glimpses of moose and bear that idly roam into our backyards and pillage our birdfeeders. There's also L.L. Bean and the Kittery Trading Post whose sporting gear advertises carefree camping, and kayaks that suggest making memories of shared excursions on the Contoocook or Merrimack Rivers.

We return, exhilarated, knowing we have breathed in enough beauty to nourish our spirits for enduring another batch of medical treatments.

DON'T

I am tired of hearing about: other people's vacations, the stock market's volatility, the cousin who lived to age 102, how a low-fat recipe is revamped, political candidates venting criticism, the vanishing of environmental protections, botched medical surgeries on your aunt or cousin.

Bitterness creeps into my lagging spirit. Long days of watchdogging and inadequate batches of shut-eye or quilting magic take their toll. Chiquita didn't keep her bananas in the refrigerator, and I don't play games of artificial cheerfulness. And don't tell me God never gives more than one can bear.

I am tired, period.

Tiredness comes in pale grays with jabs of mud brown and smears of hazardous blue, and I am easily stunted by things bright or fast moving, I am ceasing to recognize anything that smacks of normality. Do not care if tomorrow is forecast as sunny. Have not had a real vacation since '96. Then Jayne, my six-year-old grand-daughter, tells me my dress is pretty.

CONNECTING

Where are you today? You who proclaim you care so much. The truth is, I cannot express exactly why I need you.

I know. It is all so new, this unfamiliar role of home caregiving. None of us neophytes has any training; this kind of helping sounds so elementary, so childlike. Even the experts say it is learned behavior. Yes, we feel empathy now and then for those less fortunate, but when required on a regular basis to rearrange our time or to upset our budgets, we hold back. Yes, I know. Our families all have some of those head shakers and "walk-aways."

Do you remember the heartrending film about the devoted naturalist and a wary lone member of the wild animal species? The wanting to connect, the weighing of risk, the fear of getting involved lurking in the longing, as in Doris Lessing's famous story of the working girl innocently helping an elderly lady once, only to find herself drawn to years of commitment. If life has already provided us with prior relationships that felt like traps, we friends or relatives could be gun shy.

I watch an Alzheimer's caregiver on TV try to calmly explain what is missing from his own life. "It's not so much the routine," he says. "I can do that." And "it's more than a phone call. It's the knowing someone's loving presence is firmly nearby." That he is not alone.

Yes, yes.

MAIL-ORDER MEDICATIONS

Rumors tell you that mail-order medicine is the way to go. You save buckets of money and avoid endless trips to the local pharmacy.

Yes, it is at times efficient—if you remember to allow ten days for delivery service; if they do not get your order mixed up with people of the same name (there are three D. Swensons in our area), if you do not switch brands without warning, confusing you with a new color, shape and name, and if they do not have to get in touch with your doctor to verify a refill. (She's on vacation.)

When you call to change a dosage, that can be even more fun. Getting transferred from one department to another, or punching two for this or six for that is not acceptable. You get crazy. You want a real person to make things right and you want it now!

This is not even including the days of anxiously checking the mailbox for small brown packages filled with padded prescription bottles, or calling long distance to say such and such has not arrived. Of course, you get excuses and have to work at patiently reminding yourself of your own shortcomings.

Darn it.

You also forgot to make a copy of that last prescription to protect yourself against further nonsense.

AMOS II

Amos the cat is curled in a sunny spot. The far away look in his eyes broadcasts that he will soon be lulled into la-la land.

Actually, I'm mad at him.

We were not able to keep a vet's appointment because, on spotting the large green carrier, he—ears back and body low to the ground—had scooted non-stop to the attic and unreachable oblivion. That carrier triggers terrible memories for him—meaning trips to the vet to fix infected teeth, painful back-end surgeries, forced confinement.

Poor fellow!

I can identify with wanting to flee. The death of my first husband made me gun shy, too. I cannot forget the places, the suffering, and the broad range of miserable unknowns. So I, too, must accept in trust what is offered, and bravely step into the milieu of more pain and loss. It's like being put in a box to be transported back to Hades.

Amos, now back from his hideaway, seeks love. He jumps onto my desk papers to sit before me, still swishing his tail a bit in discomfiture, but relinquishing , according to his eyes convey an entreaty for forgiveness.

WORRIES

While doing the everyday mundane things like cooking and dressing, I worry. As a woman I simply think about my future. I will sell the big house because I will no longer need it or be able to afford it. But where will I be living? Be dependent? Me?

I cannot categorize the worries. Perhaps my condition has a name . . . like anxiety syndrome or post traumatic stress disorder . . . .

I must remember that many Psalms begin with whines and worries and end with a strange but jubilant kind of rejoicing.

I must remind myself of the adage that when the pupil is ready, the teacher will appear.

In particular, I remember that I worried about David finding a compassionate minister with whom he could easily relate during the difficult times ahead. And PRESTO, our new associate minister, Reverend Jim Pirie appeared. Warm, open to the concerns of ill people, experienced working with the over sixty crowd, *and* raised in the granite business!

SOCKS

Even my view of socks has changed.

Once it was children's stray ones hidden under the bed, or sissy knee socks, or argyles carefully knitted in resounding colors. Now, singles in dark messy drawers are no longer looked upon as traumatic. Memories of status rules about them are almost funny.

Because David's feet are cold all the time, socks are essential. He always likes a certain kind of lightweight wool, never polyester. And he always likes to wash his own, stretching them on antique metal frames to hang by the shower curtain, reminiscent of early times before automatic washers and electric dryers. The clean heavy woolen ski socks in Scandinavian designs lie tucked, unused, in the back of the dresser drawer.

Now he needs elastic knee-highs for swollen ankles. So I traipse to stores to find just the right ones. Places like T.J. Maxx and Marshalls do not cater to his wants. I check catalogs, and the medical sections of pharmacies. No luck. Closing my eyes to cost, I eventually find them in the Vermont Country Store catalog. I order them.

Hallelujah!

KEPT

I've decided I am a kept woman.

"Kept" in history meant champagne and pearls with an aura of blatant sexuality.

What I mean here is, there are those who care about me.

Now, my daughter keeps me in colorful quilting sketch pads for my random ideas as to future quilt projects.

My friends keep me in books about matters of shared interest, knowing a good read passed palm to palm means a cup of cold water to a mighty thirsty woman.

My God keeps me in supplies of epiphanies, those surprising out-of-context events and changes, reminding me that, as the hymn says, there is a wideness in God's mercy.

Some may believe that those subtle gifts are only coincidences. But I believe in what author Lynn Huber shares in her *Revelations on the Road*. "A coincidence is a miracle in which God wishes to remain anonymous."

REMISSION

The latest checkup suggests we are in remission. (That's not transmission as in cars or submission as in alpha and omega wolf dominance. It means that the dreaded disease has at least temporarily halted its spreading accompanied by possible healing.)

We do not know how to receive this good news. We have been walking the treadmill of good behavior so diligently for so long that we seem unable to be jubilant. Why are we prepared for only the worst? Though always hoping and praying for the miraculous, we do not know how to accept such news. When it finally registers, we quickly turn objective.

Our three-floor farmhouse living is now burdensome. There is no bedroom or full bath on the first floor, and we now pay exorbitant taxes and yard-keeping fees. So we begin to agonize over the possibility of selling a home we adore. Could we easily find a one-story ranch to supply our present needs? Would I, alone, have the energy to do all that needs to be done? All in the uncertain time period that would coincide with David's plateau of remission?

The answer is no, but it does not stop us rugged New Hampshirites.

After calling a friendly neighbor who is a realtor, we discuss the possible course before us, and I begin the property search for a smaller place.

It is midwinter and my days spin out into a measureless length.

MOVING I

Good sense is derailed temporarily as price and profit take over our usual emphasis on declining health issues. In simple terms, our value system temporarily runs amuck.

How do you price a house where memories abound that defy logical evaluation? Where you remember wallpapering the hall with that colorful bird/flower print? Where the grandchildren decorated the tall tree in the front corner by the old fireplace? Where your husband masterfully installed stately granite entry posts? Where you bathed in a footed Victorian tub? Ordered the gazebo from the Concord prison system? Where you planted Laurie's lilacs, and blew out Bill's happy birthday candles?

Price it too high and no one will buy. Price it too low, and we will be the ones to cry. In a world where we accuse others of corporate greed, we find ourselves not exhibiting modest principles so often claimed.

RETREATING

I must be exhibiting undue signs of stress because my friend Ellen gives me a flier about a nifty place here in our state to go on a personal retreat. She highly recommends it, and points to the many possible programs offered. Seen as a relief from the daily scanning of properties sounds appealing, as does the chance to escape constant medical issues and household drudgeries, I study the offerings and choose one that will focus on the arts, body movement, and labyrinth walking. As I am still able to leave David during the day, it sounds surprisingly feasible.

The popularity of brief retreats these days points to the reality of needed escape hatches. Old concepts of stuffy rigid, pious retreats have been replaced by new designs that include happy hour and introductions to new art forms. Everyone—from the newly married, the recently divorced, the stressed-out business executive—now knows that there are special places that can provide a release from a daily routine, and a reacquaintance or reconnecting with the inner dilemma of a spacious self.

We all need to retreat from pettiness, stupid habits, others' undue expectations.

Bless the Catholic sisters who often provide these restful places.

WHEELCHAIRS

Walmart probably does not sell wheelchairs.

The doctor has given me a written slip authorizing a wheelchair rental because David's difficulty getting from room to room has increased.

Did you know that medical supply houses are not on every corner? I finally proceed to a given address of a medical supply house.

The clerks are grand. Sensing my stupidity about disability they quickly teach me a few bare facts. I can't lift the regular size chair and the light one is a modern day marvel that comes in a variety of colors. They are not instantly in stock like canned tomatoes or 100 watt lightbulbs. It seems they are individually ordered or must be brought in from some faraway warehouse.

David's concern about pneumatic tires (which once graced his father's early design) is quickly ignored. The new jobs have a tough new substance that defies definition and excites marvel in contemporary ingenuity. With doorways to measure, I note the size of seats, wonder about furniture arrangements. I return home feeling like a confident, modern woman who has just passed her math exam, only to hear David announce that no wife of his is going to have to push him around.

BRIDGE

A bridge game to me is simply a few hours out with friends, but I have learned that it is also in a sense a lesson in forgiveness.

When I first started to play the game, I would return home only to lie awake nights reviewing the hands, in particular recalling what I considered my unforgivable mistakes. How could they stand it! Why did I play that jack instead of that king? Then, in my mind's review, there were the times when my partner of the round had done something stupid, preventing us from getting that 700 rubber.

Now, as a seasoned player, I am able to play with certain friends, knowing with assurance that we all make mistakes but we tend to only momentarily experience regret. Then we move on. We know it's only a game; we express a universal kind of acceptance. We all have good and bad days, meaning lapses of recollection regarding standard rules, and the risk of which cards will be dealt, and how the distribution will fall.

Isn't that like life? Eventually realization comes that I can usually forgive others before I can forgive myself. There are always contributing factors that soften the game.

GARAGE SALE

Although our house hasn't sold, I decide to start with a quick garage sale—except that I discover there is no such thing. It takes hours to sort our drawers and closets for discards. I get bogged down in rediscovering that odd gift from the past and reading that term paper written in 1957. The handling and reevaluation of such detailed things is emotionally exhausting, not to speak of the physical effort of lugging stuff in bags and boxes out to the piles in our two-car garage. Then there is the pricing, the heat, the need for display tables, the arranging, the finding of helpers. It becomes easy to sputter and gripe.

It rains on the first advertised date. Ditto on the second, though a few brave souls wander in and buy things like a damaged table and a box of party favors from 1989. So, with the help of Patty, my nephew's wife, I re-sort and haul what is left to Goodwill and an upcoming group rummage sale.

The profit, which is supposed to be enough to cover moving costs, is only enough to re-upholster two living room chairs.

Downsizing usually refers to job cutting methods. Reducing refers to overweight persons. For us, discarding means letting go of stuff that obstructs and clutters the deepest of feelings.

It is never too late.

What I prize may not be what I thought it would be.

TV

I seek rest and TV gives: the weather in San Francisco, a segment on magnified ant life, the Durham school board minutes, a program on transvestite American males, a sitcom with canned laughter and a trite story line, the real life heartbreak of a teen missing persons case, a hard sell channel pushing a flashy outfit for only 3 easy payments, people competing for $50,000 by seeing who can eat the most worms, and a repeat broadcast of last week's congressional hearing on a scandal.

It lets me down.

I must find solace in some other place.

OUT AND ABOUT

David still wants to be out and about as much as possible. He does not mind wearing oxygen tubes in public, or lugging a small oxygen canister. I admire him for his positive attitude and ask myself if I could be carefree about the stares regarding nonconformity? Would I as a woman be more self-conscious? Would I feel forced to stay home?

If we enter a restaurant, we get more than a single glance. Do we invade their sense of privacy? Interrupt their illusions about perfect functioning body parts? Destroy their enjoyment of a shrimp cocktail or an expensive night on the town with the sight of a handsome man gasping for air?

Breathing is something we all take for granted. Yet it often takes the breathing difficulties of a friend or loved one to open our eyes. I know I have become more conscious of the woman with the small tank in her grocery basket, or the man trying to load his folding chair into the car.

Three cheers for the sensitive people who have championed those with disabilities as they seek equal rights for those with conditions that demand wheelchairs, walkers, oxygen paraphernalia, and other life-support systems.

OFFICE MESSES

Today we start to sort David's home office, a large renovated space over the kitchen. It is filled to capacity with wooden file cabinets, dusty geology reference books, stone samples carefully marked, mailing supplies, job records in manila packets, GS maps, a drafting board, a Savin copier, his father's carved walnut desk, a fax machine. The tabulation goes on and on.

It is a daunting task, and later we are surprised to learn from Guy (his water-geologist nephew) that much of what David had laboriously collected over a lifetime is now available via modern technology.

David's knowledge of the granite world is incredible, his expertise once referenced in *The Wall Street Journal*. His advice and good sense were sought by architects and curious laymen. While he excels at keeping detailed records, the lilt of joy in his voice on sharing information gratis is a pure delight to hear.

But sorting out one's life before death is exhausting. By 2 p.m. he ate his yogurt and fell into bed, laughing in remembrance of the Yale classmate who had said in disbelief, "You're going to make a living from rocks?"

VIEWS OF SICKNESS

Each segment of my life seems to reveal a different view of the medical world. As a child it was Band-Aids, coughs requiring red syrupy suppressants, acne, whispers of mono, and an uncle who had lumbago. What was *that*? Then it was facts about menstrual cycles, the experience of childbirth, and the alarming distinction between a rectal and an oral thermometer.

Midlife led me to an awareness of jet lag, penicillin, diabetes, x-rays, and the importance of vitamins and dietary supplements. Only gradually did it dawn on me that one could be sick and not be in bed.

Somewhere in there I began to hear about diuretics, liquid Band-Aids, chemo, melanoma, cholesterol, Parkinson's, emphysema, and really unpleasant reference to bronchial dilators, incontinence, irritable bowel syndrome, with the surprising news that staples are used in surgery, broken leg bandages can get wet, and tiny cameras can now be swallowed. Even some conditions of age are being redefined, while TV ads blare about hemorrhoids and Viagra.

Now I brace for the curiously named conditions as well as the newly invented highly advertised medications.

RESPONSIBILITIES

I announce to David that I better start taking over the bills. It has been a long time for me—since the 1980s to be exact. He had always liked to do it, a Harvard MBA who enjoyed chasing pennies and totaling columns while I, on the other hand, am not good at anything mathematical.

The first day, devising my own rudimentary way, I sort the statements, highlight budgetary concerns and soon come to the stark realization that times have drastically changed. I gasp at the cost of heating oil, the cost of gas needed to keep two cars on the road, and the dizzying record of various medical expenses. All those years he had protected me from financial worry. How could I have been so lucky?

Later, when I casually ask for his help with a puzzling telephone bill, his willingness is hampered by an inability to focus, and the invoice sits untouched by his blue plaid chair. It is days before I realize that he is no longer able to deal with such things; that his mental processes have permanently broken down or disappeared.

What feels like a burden of total responsibility sinks in with a colossal thud, becoming alarmingly immediate and terribly precise.

MANTRAS

Memorized short verses learned in childhood now have a way of silently springing back, unexpectedly, into my life as I sit by his side, dash from A to B, or rush to get things done. Phrases like "God's mercy endureth forever" and "Take no thought of the morrow." The language of yesterday applies to today's key experiences.

Is it mind control? Parents' obsessions? A sign of one's values, bottle fed along with the oatmeal and the prune juice?

The truth is, my phrases are not all biblical. Mixed in with the mantras may be a swear word, or a verse from a musical, like "Love changes things." After "Lord have mercy, Christ have mercy" may be my hearty rendition of "Goodnight, My Darling, Goodnight, My Love." I use whatever alters the moment.

The Bible does incite wonderful heartfelt instruction. "Let not your heart be troubled," "I am the Way," and "Send the Holy Spirit into our hearts to direct and rule us according to your will" are wonderfully soothing. Maybe that last one actually came from the *Book of Common Prayer*.

Today I settle down to quilt to the tune of "underneath are the everlasting arms."

WAITING ROOM II

Today I sit in a Stephen King kind of waiting room. Yes, I'm thinking of the author's ability to describe humans in certain situations as monstrous specimens. Unreal and nameless souls in a medical world that at times feels grotesque.

Some of my impressions are unfairly fed by random observation: the ratty sneakers; the grubby, soiled jacket; the hats and scarves that hide chemo-induced baldness. And the overheard unintelligible gibberish uttered between non-English-speaking couples; the loud, doting, too friendly next of kin; the overweight matron in the soiled housedress being carefully watchdogged by the stylish immaculate daughter. And not just the socks in sandals and the faithful but pasty-complexioned spouse, but the colorlessness of the place, add to the overall surrealistic, outer space effect.

The sudden flashback of another confused soul who once sat beside me in a Boston hospital clutching a live sparrow, hidden from view within her tatty bag, causes me to dash from this oppressive waiting room.

We caregivers come out of our dens of fear, ignorance, and undusted homes for just a short time, brought together by ceaseless, unquestioning demands. Not wanting to view or to be viewed, but acutely aware of feeling so responsible for our loved ones, we make up the odd-lot communion of cynical and weary survivalists.

It is only the presence of a delicate but wiggly child with long shining angelic blond curls that causes many of us tired warriors to smile in spite of ourselves.

SURVIVAL KIT

What is a survival kit?

Before cancer diagnosis it was a Boy Scout pocketknife, rain gear, dry socks, matches, and an energy bar. After cancer it is medications, faith, a urinal, and sufficient medical insurance.

Before September 11 it was an attitude of "I will live forever." After September 11 it is shocking new daily awareness, a renewed appreciation of what is precious, an elective review of what we had learned and forgotten in chapter and verse from the lives of others.

Survival kit? That's too small an image.

Valise? That's too bulky and old-fashioned.

We have graduated to backpacks complete with cell phone to alert the forest ranger when we slip off the trail.

Then again, there's the waterproof canvas type, light but floppy, and the duffle bag meant for camp and army life.

In childhood we played the game "I packed my suitcase" as we were challenged to remember all the contents of others' bags. These were usually a long list of crazy and improbable things. Who can forget Grandma singing a song about "packing up your troubles in an old kit bag?"

Will *we* ever be able to declare the most important element for life's hazardous journey? Who is the ranger in your life?

DOWN

Watching the slowing down of David's body functions is heartbreaking. I compare this month to the same time last year. The change is gradual, the evidence lurking in decreasing appetite and an awareness of atrophy in his upper leg muscles.

Silent ponderings, only, accompany daily restrictions. Will this be his Yale classmate's last visit? What kind of aid is out there that will assist his getting around?

Being emotionally "down" is seldom discussed. It is denied. Coming down with measles meant a certain number of days with spots. But cancer?

There is definitely an increased weakness. Walking from the car to the door takes longer. He does not admit it or talk about it. The day is mostly filled with naps and regimented medical procedures. Increased dosages of prednisone give his face a square jaw kind of filling out, his hands a mysterious series of dark blotchy markings.

Downhill skiing suggests speed, but this snail-paced downhill of cancer requires patience, vigilance, and periodic embraces.

We grew up with the phrase "down and out." Was there an "up and in?"

YESTERDAYS II

Was there ever another life, "before?" What was it like? Were we once carefree? When we laughed, swam, or hiked together—his breathing normal, his handsome face healthy and alert—did we foolishly just take our freedom for granted?

Was there really a time when we jumped wildly into bed, when we happily traveled, racing to retrieve the beat-up suitcase from the luggage carousel after the adventurous journey? Attended upbeat concerts, reverently sat in places together, relaxed side by side?

What happened to yesterday, to passion, to a partnership of equals?

The days, months, and years of treatments and gobbled energy were filled with Tuesday oxygen deliveries, charting of pills, frantic tiredness, figuring the best way to adjust to frightening things.

Please God.

I do not want to forget the best as I slog through this horror of watching him silently struggle to just stay alive.

HOUSES

I find a house that could fulfill our needs. A large ranch with a small lot, and we find the courage to make an offer here in our scenic tax-free but inflated real estate market. The bid is accepted, with the clause that we must first sell our rambling old house. They call it a contingency clause.

More pressure is on.

I lie awake nights now for more than one reason.

With high hopes, our house is shown to endless potential buyers, which requires a lot of neatening up on my part, and lots of last-minute shoving and hiding of stray items into forgotten places. Cleaning up is a routine that gets ridiculously tiring. Even the cat learns to disappear when he sees me rushing about.

Sometimes I stop and stare and suck in the effect of my high-grade (ha) taste in color and design, privately treasuring my garage sale antiques and collectibles hanging out in the neatened-up space. I say, "Wow" out loud as we rush to disappear before the arrival of the scheduled potential buyer.

Houses reflect who we are—our strengths and weaknesses, our preferences, our fervent nesting habits all a naked revelation.

As I grab the garbage—no time to package it properly so we take it with us—we say we could live anywhere, but we admit a deep attachment to this gracious old lady.

HOSPITAL RENOVATION

The hospital is undergoing its own change, so the return to the hospital after a period of remission means additional adjustments. They're enlarging the cancer center. Our visits become another maze of uncertainty, bordered by new brick and seamless glass.

It is good to know they will enlarge some of these cubbyhole places, but some of us, like family pets, prefer the spaces to stay the same.

There are a lot of temporary locations and a new outpatient entrance. (The front is the back, the back now the front.) Where do I park? I enter the wrong entrance and push the wheelchair for what feels like the width of Lake Winnipesaukee. Men in construction hats and heavy equipment have joined the nurses looking busy, running back and forth, creating additional confusion.

The return brings friendly greetings from some of the same cheery faces and there are aides standing around wanting to be helpful.

The hospital is always a place of routine business for some, but it's a grand citadel of hope to those of us treading through the last days with our courageous loved ones.

REJECTION

We are feeling rejected.

We have revealed ourselves to numerous prospective buyers who have trooped through our private space, invading our closets and cubbyholes. I guess they don't like our paisley wallpaper in the bedroom, our choice of a simple country kitchen, our painting of the young girl at the beach. You can see I have internalized our frustrating summer.

The cat Amos gets left in the basement during the showings. He likes it down there with its glimmer of mice, and the small windows that provide close-up views of birds hiding in the grass, but he tires of the dark change of menu and eventually yaks impatiently to be allowed back up, cobwebs dangling from his handsome whiskers.

While I know that Durham taxes and Route 4 traffic noise are probably what cancelled an easy sell, I hang in there even though David is due another battery of tests.

ANDY

David's brother Andy invited a large array of friends and relatives to celebrate his birthday yesterday afternoon at the family beach house. It was a festive but informal affair, catered, outdoors, under tents, complete with hearty toasts and family engendered music.

David had looked forward to the get-together, especially to the arrival of relatives from California and Washington, DC. But he found the festivities draining, and as the sun went down and the crowds dwindled, he silently made his way across the lawn to the house to stretch out on the ancient green porch swing.

A few of us quietly gathered around, propping ourselves on the motley mix of peeling porch chairs. Someone started a tune, someone else softly joined in, and soon he was surrounded by the purr of gentle rounds and old ditties out of our diverse yet common pasts.

In the interludes of quiet, time actually stood still.

Bathed in the heat of the summer and the gentle hum of loved ones, he dozed, our love for him soothing the fleeting moments.

The long, narrow porch with its chipped gray painted floor that I had scrubbed so often with sweat dripping, became the place where we watchers became the holy ones.

LAYERS

During the last ten years I have been designing and leading workshops on the spirituality of aging for churches and other organizations. On introducing the various concepts of life stages, it usually becomes clear that the view of our lives midlife and beyond has been ignored or trivialized. It is often through art forms that we reveal truths and changes about ourselves, so I often use a cross-section of a geode. It is an impressive artifact in many shades of blue, with a center core of deep color bordered by various shadings that speak about time frames, stability, and even beauty.

Layers. While it is already familiar and trendy to layer clothes, for me there is now the new awareness of layers of faith because I am digging deeper as David's body weakens. The first layer is easy—the responses taught and almost automatic. But what is the second layer? Obstacles as new choices?

"Live in the layers" the poets continue their message as I struggle with the BLTs of caregiver routines—the spiritually nutritious sandwich of the daily, mysterious, difficult, changed, gratifying, hidden.

DEATH II

Words about death are raining on me in puzzling bunches. Go away. Go away. "Pass on," "kick the bucket," "the deceased." Corpse is used only in detective stories. We speak in riddles and rhymes, with words a cover-up for unbearable things.

One person says we need closure and not with doors. Another writer coins the phrase "rendezvous with death," implying that we will rejoin a loved one in the sweet by-and-by. Another says there is a picturesque Rainbow Bridge where we will again meet our departed furry friend. Old words like "quagmire" and "slough of despond" are counterpoint to today's injunction to simply "work it out." Mixed signals of let it all hang out or don't cry have a way of confusing the issue when I want to squawk and wail while my life, like the heavy machine, goes into reverse gear.

I struggle with where God is in today's jargon.

As I make a stab at evaluating death, I cling to and fall back on old promises. As in the familiarity of "Precious is the death of his Godly ones" and the comfort of "passed out of death into Life."

LEGACIES

Others' real life stories continue to give me strength.

When my niece Pam's husband died he left her a complicated sprinkler system with an unknown code. Laughing into the sporadic spray, she and a neighbor took a whole day to figure it out by trial and error.

Rena cares for a paralyzed husband at home. She has done so for nine years.

Ann cares not only for a sick husband but a ninety-seven-year-old mother, yet she also finds ways to feed herself. She knows how to get away for brief canoe trips or theatre outings in New York City.

When Ethel's husband died in his sleep on a train going west to visit their daughter, she crawled into the upper birth to try to give him artificial respiration.

These are not the kinds of stories that make the headlines. So often we use the word "strength" to refer only to physical stamina—miles jogged, cycled, or climbed. While these traits are noteworthy, too often we neglect the value of interior qualities of perseverance, compassion, and humor.

Additional revelation: Those who save others may die shortly thereafter. The man who dug the first air hole for the Pennsylvania miners committed suicide. And the man who rescued baby Jessica from the Texas oil well shot himself.

ADMITTING NEEDS

Friends' concerns that I am trying to be wonder woman comes as a surprise to me. They ask, "When are you taking a break?" "Who in your family checks in regularly?" "Have you asked his PCP about all those oxygen worries?"

The five of us meet once a month to privately hash over basic issues experienced by all older women but ignored by everyone else. It has been a haven of support for years, and now an exercise in stark reality when they insist I act out a response.

Today they gave me an assignment to be completed before our next monthly meeting. I must ask someone for some particular kind of help. They volunteered to be my guinea pigs as I practice admitting and voicing specific needs aloud to family and friends. This exercise is presented with kindness, and with a warning that they may be brutally honest and refuse or suggest some other sort of negotiation.

I agree to the exercise, and ask friends Fin and Joyce if they could help me pack for the eventual move. After three phone calls to find a date that is agreeable, we start to pack the big set of white china with the gold trim. This is a new experience, sharing the job, as I have moved many times and always done my own packing. It is not easy to see them industriously wrapping things up. I do not like to see them work. Am I afraid of losing their friendship? Because I'm worrying about them doing too much, we take a lengthy break, falling into comfy chairs to chat in delight about the unexpected sight of five wild turkeys that congregate under the kitchen bird feeder!

NOT DRIVING

Is there anything more threatening to a man than telling him he can no longer drive? No matter who gets to say it—a doctor, wife, faithful friend—such news strikes lethal dismay in the heart of the victim. Actually, rage is a better word.

David and I have our first real argument in sixteen years.

The car appears to be a symbol of privilege and freedom. Just idly sitting there in the garage or driveway, it declares itself to be the always available friend. More than transportation, it signifies the endless ability to be in charge, to choose preferred directions, routes, and unlimited destinations. Power in a metallic body.

Now, dependency fears, usually in disguise, jump to the surface and explode. Reassurances that faithful friends promise to tote him about fall on deaf ears. Reference to passenger safety has absolutely no significance. Acceptance of another loss is just too galling.

Behind the wheel is where David has always been and where he prefers to be now. Sick or well. Meant to be.

Strategy: Let some neutral magician give the official word.

TRUTH TELLING

Who will be there for me when I cannot drive the car, negotiate the supermarket, and adjust my baggy stocking as it slips embarrassingly down in public?

Today I allow such painful thoughts to surface.

I picture a gray old lady struggling to get out of her lumpy chair, there in her dingy apartment, where only dust and self-pity congregate.

I know.

Self-pity is a terrible thing. People would say "Don't be silly, Harriet. You have children who will."

What? Tell me!

My mother was as mad as a hornet when Dad died. She had told us repeatedly she wanted to go first. Now I understand. Extended living alone might feel more like a curse than a blessing.

The good news for all of us today seems to be that significant others now come in all shapes and sizes, not just as spouses or blood-related next of kin. There is a widening circle of understanding that has moved beyond immediate family to neighbor, local church, partner, and global friend.

I am brought back to the basic issue of loving well.

NO SELL

We are not able to sell the big house during the summer. We take it off the market.

I am disappointed, to put it mildly, and feel like weeks of mind numbing daily straightening have come to naught. Now I must face another winter caregiving in our huge, charming but inconvenient home.

I try to accept the philosophy that it was meant to be, so easily voiced by those who try to be comforting. But the idea that someone stronger and smarter than I has determined what is best for us is impossible to swallow. Proverbial advice provides little comfort, and is as raw as the squeaky wrench of chalk on a blackboard. God's hand in everybody's business? Just bad luck! Mind over matter? When a door closes, a window opens.

But I do take friend Kathy's advice to bury a small statue of St. Joseph upside down in the backyard for luck, believing that we could now easily flounder financially as I sadly watch David continue to weaken physically.

THE GREAT ESCAPE

It is really a fishing camp. In contrast to the rollicking round of activities at the family beachhouse, this is a peaceful sanctuary. Every September for two weeks we leave the world behind. For David, it means change from closed-in interiors to wide expanses of sky and the freshest of air. For me, it is a form of salvation.

We have told few people where it is. Just two hours north, hidden among stately pines, this tiny rented spot sits at the end of a winding dirt driveway, its screened porch facing one of New Hampshire's many charming small lakes.

The basics include a private beach, an indoor bathroom and electricity, and bottled drinking water that can be easily hauled from nearby. As I was familiar with real down-to-earth camping with my first husband, this spot seems luxurious.

And it is here that I really see the progression of David's condition: from active swimming to counted foot steps back and forth on the beach—his carved walking stick in hand, his small oxygen tank in his backpack—in his slowed gait of minimally getting around. I no longer run the oxygen through the window to the liquid tank on the back of the truck. Instead, the owner of the camp helps me move the compressor onto the porch. I know this is to be our last precious time together in our magical spot.

This year everything will be up to me—the advance cooking, the choice of reading and music, the preordering of adequate meds, the car loading. It is a fierce exercise of logistics. I pack ten carry-all bags, not suitcases, as I will be carrying all the bedding and the food. I try to do advance planning, but the actual departure time runs much later than planned, by the time I pack the perishables and gas up the car.

The first night we have pre-made meatloaf sandwiches, one of David's favorites. But I am so exhausted that I fear I have made a mistake as to my own physical and emotional limits.

But each new day promises nature's sights and sounds, even from the small kitchen window over the sink. A meditative renewal takes place as we get pampered by signs of God's presence.

The first day I guide David outdoors to bask under the mammoth trees. The forty-foot pines in our cove spread their protective sentinel-like branches while two immense birches guard us on the left. Shimmering leaves from the slender beech trees hum their overture of harmonious murmurs. To the right a kingfisher may expertly dive for dinner or a white butterfly may flaunt her fragile beauty in the sun. The float, moored 30 feet off shore, idly rocks in the late morning breezes. Sitting in the broad bowl of silence, we can simmer in satisfaction, be astonished by the momentary sense of peace, and stillness, absorb the warmth, feel joined forever.

David can easily doze; a grasshopper may brush his arm; a soft caterpillar drop without warning onto our bare feet. Hello!

I always look forward to hearing the loons, and once during a brief afternoon swim experienced one close by me in the water. David, sprawled in the oversized beach chair, marveled at the sight, and bragged many times to his buddies about it. For me, the glow of that shared loveliness still astounds me. These large black and white birds are often categorized by others as "eerie and sad," as if from nonsense choruses from Gilbert and Sullivan. Out there in the dark, their trembling calls—a piercing reminder of hope—dependable, always welcome, surprising me with their sporadic, uninvited message.

It makes me feel as if I have waded with eternal things.

Then there was the time the seagull appeared, his whiteness out of place in an inland location of soft green and brown, not coastal rock and sky blue oceanic horizon. He stopped and rested on our rocking raft. He appeared three days running, so I suggested he had settled in with—what? a wild goose? a compromised duck? And of course, my philosophical whimsy went to work. If he wasn't lost, is it possible he is smart? Had discovered some advantage for him here? With God giving us so many conundrums, I tie the thought to illness. David's diagnosis could be wrong. The gull labeled as stupid may just be adventurous. Are we likewise able to explore new avenues of treatment?

We hear about 911 from the owner while we are here, and drive in to town to a small white steepled church on a hill to join the locales in prayers of entreaty.

Sometimes my Quaker friend Edith from a neighboring lake drops in, or David's friend Roger brings his own sandwich and tidbits of local politics.

Sometimes we briefly leave the premises to drive on short scenic excursions, dropping in on Steve and Sally Swenson in Conway, and stopping at a dog show—David's first. We do not shop much for tourist temptations and seldom eat out, preferring to hasten back to our leisurely suppers on our porch. Here we can enjoy hearing the simple dip of a canoe paddle, uninterrupted conversation, watch the sunset, and declare that everything tastes better here. Once we talked about our parents, pondering why they had married, aware of their differences in temperament, background, and ideas about frugality. We reviewed that we both had short mothers and businesslike fathers. Mine was a Maine townie who became a building estimator; his was a hard-working Swedish quarry owner fostering a family granite business, which has survived four generations.

A key moment for both couples seems to have been the arrival of the radio and TV into their mundane lives. TV watching was allowed only for a smiling piano player or a Red Sox game. Our parents gave us ice cream on Sunday and bought us shoes at places where we could see our toes in the funny X-ray machine. At our wedding we had chosen to have each parent (though long deceased) to be reverently named by the clergy. The camp is always a special place for reminiscence, where time stands still and everyday things wait.

Once I found a lone duck with a broken wing, by the water's edge. He had preened, pretended nonchalance, testing me out with his sporadic approaches, and—after his quick grabs at gentle handouts—eventually, lakeside, fell asleep propped on one leg, his head resting, screwed 180 degrees west, onto his own soft, dark pillow of down. He appeared vulnerable as he napped, so I decided I could not leave. A stray cat or a slinking weasel could attack. So my usual schedule of swimming before dinner preparation that day was cancelled. I watched in silence as he slept on. For him, rest meant relief from fears of natural predators. Rest for me meant reduction of swollen ankles and escape from anxious cerebral thought about my mate's deteriorating condition.

Always cycles of caring amidst the lives of God's creatures!

We were once at the cabin during a major hurricane. The power went out, but we still had food, a gas stove, and the lake for washing. When a giant pine fell, blocking our driveway, we trusted the owner to rescue us, and before long two rugged men in jeans and work boots appeared with a power saw to open up the road.

That day, in gray light, I remember how I sat by the window in full view of the angry turmoil of churning waters, finding confidence and serenity in the simplest of handiwork. At night, we snuggled while the wind howled. Unafraid, we refused to worry about the amount of liquid oxygen left.

At the end of our stay, we went back to pick up the cat at the nice place that caters to spoiled felines—a place with air conditioning, color-coordinated private rooms, soft afghans, and window seats. (We are always told that Amos is a talker. We already knew that.)

On paying the bill for the deluxe accommodations, we hear his feeble complaints from the rear of the car, behind the oxygen cylinders, the dirty laundry, and the mix of gear.

As he exits the confining green carrier on arrival home, he remembers his whereabouts and skulks hastily to his usual dining corner. Empty of course. So I gladly fulfill his wish for a little tuna, as I am glad to be again under the orders of my furry friend as we return to our big, rambling, unsold house.

LISTENING

I admit I sometimes have trouble slowing down enough to really hear the inner pulse of David's life revealed before me. I've learned that the cancer patient can talk about difficult issues only when he/she feels able, which to the caregiver may not feel like the best time. He may choose to do so after a brief rest or in an unplanned moment. This requires me to be willing to talk one-on-one in spite of the interruption of my usual schedule. Although Deborah Tannen, who writes about gender differences in communication, says that women are the ones who most often take the role of listener, I think that both of us do pay close attention, but neither of us is in the habit of chattering about minor details on any subject.

Today it is David who hears a painful message and gives in to the vet's insistence to euthanize his dog. Our drive to Stratham is a solemn one, and I am the one to sob uncontrollably as Cecil ceases to move. I am the one who screams, "Why aren't you the one crying?" as David, stoically sitting on the hard cubicle bench, takes his silent but loving turn doing the listening, the paying attention, the letting go.

PANIC

I impatiently say to David one night "talk to me."

As we sit at home in our favorite chairs reading, immobilized before a TV program rambling on about inconsequential escapades of others, I am jarred into a stark new realization of my own increased emotional aloneness. While the cancer cells are doing their own kind of business, taking over his brain as well as his lungs and liver, my level of awareness has taken a new hit. There is a sudden new knowledge that we have had few recent and real mental exchanges lately. There have been too many nights of visual proximity without communication. Yes, shared silence had always been a rich part of our marriage, but the pain of too much stillness is forcing the stillness of death.

The realization of such loss gives me a jab of panic. Is his ability to be totally present with me to be gone forever?

So I begin the grieving process while he is still with me, an abrupt reminder of what the future will be like.

To live without him? Never.

"What, never?"

"No never!"

CONDO

The loss of the chosen ranch to another buyer and the shocking late sale of our unlisted house requires some hasty rushing around to again view what is easily available in the area. Did Kathy's bizarre suggestion to plant the St. Joseph figurine upside down in the backyard really work?

I find a corner unit in a Durham complex of six condos. Except for the new white carpeting, I find it alluring with its view of trees and pond. Its best feature is a sunny corner bedroom for David. A small deck opens off the bedroom, promising good light and the possibility of a screened porch come spring.

I sense a feeling of rightness, though the idea of such restricted living after the large, roomy high-ceilinged farmhouse keeps me from making an immediate decision, as does the disappointment that I could not handle a large dog there. Knowing friends in the area helps me take the step. I make out the binder check and return to wide-awake midnight envisioning of bookcase placement, couch fitting, excess quilting paraphernalia, and the necessity of cleaning the dark, overstuffed basement in the old place.

The condo will include a plowed driveway, a mowed lawn, an attached garage, and a corner fireplace, all of which tell me that the decision is probably the best for us right now.

STUFF

The unexpected opportunity to quickly sell the farmhouse prompts the need to rent a storage unit. So David rides with me as we spend an entire Saturday tracking down facilities in various adjacent towns.

He jots down the information as to place, price, and size of various units before we decide on a Dover storage facility, clean and convenient, with a six-month limit to this kind of financial expense.

I lie awake some more. Like any move, I visualize our furniture. What will be kept? What will the children want? What should be stored? My attachment to several family antiques interferes with decision-making, so I call a few dealers to get consignment rates and consider what could go to Goodwill. Then I begin to make short strategic trips to the storage unit with the endless small boxes of things to be needed later. An emptying out, an overdue.

Where had it all come from? When did clutter and surplus ever guarantee us happiness? I am reminded of the man who on the death of his wife simply walked out the front door never to return.

I later find David's notes of that busy day. They are illegible. His wanting to help and his covert hiding of his inability to do so poignantly and tearfully bring back that day we had in togetherness.

ACCEPTANCE

We return to the same gray hospital room for another office visit.

When it sinks in what the blue-coated oncologist in well-shined loafers is saying and not saying—with casual reference to "spreading" and "easing of testing" David and I enter a new place all our own. In riveting English, we are out of remission.

The fuzzy pronouncement and medical gibberish hover wickedly in the air.

That's it?

Stricken, frantic thoughts afloat yet frozen. The shock weighs us down. Any audible responses evaporate. Efforts to voice and discuss the issue become strangely otherworldly. It has come to this? A massive wall slammed down upon the still living, the still blindly hopeful?

We feel betrayed.

Where is God?

Does failure of modern-day medicine demand more from us than we have already given?

Knowledge of stages of grief according to the Kübler-Ross model does not bring consolation. I reach out to embrace David, who is trying to digest this latest blast of terminal news. I see the same look he had on the day his dog died. I watch him watching a favorite doctor, his icon, his bastion of hope, as well as his own grueling contest for his future all go crashing to the unfriendly floor.

No sympathy is expressed by the so-called professional.

DEATH III

When folks tell me that losses always come in threes, I cringe. It is not helpful. We all know there are serial killers. But serial deaths?

Yes, I know death has always been around. Bored children in backseat car games grew up believing that cemeteries just meant ten points in a counting game, and adult agony over loss can be a warning about future attachments, causing doubt as to the sanity of daring to love again.

But those caring for someone who can no longer speak know that waves of loving still pass between them. They know that love is stronger than death.

HOSPICE CARE

I find some help in the form of hospice care (Once a doctor has admitted that a cure is no longer possible, the patient and family can choose to be cared for at home with loved ones based on the medical assumption that the patient has six months or less to live.)

I made the contact, and the hospice team arrived, skilled at immediately putting anxious families and patients at ease. I will never forget that day.

We talked in the living room, with David and I both amazed. These people spoke our language about the kinds of things that are really going on at our house: the sundry fears, the availability of pain medication, the many specific ways they will be able to help us in the future. They really listen. They give direct answers.

A physical therapist will show David and me about dealing with falls. A nurse will appear regularly to monitor medicine and feelings. A respite volunteer will provide free time for my errands. An aide will attend to his hygiene needs. His comfort will be foremost.

Praise God!

FALLING

David fell last night.

The loud thud heard from downstairs was terrifying.

His leg had buckled as he left our upstairs bathroom, and I raced up to find him on the floor of his office. The look on his face was a kind of mortification. The inability to get up, on discovering such weakness, was impossible for him to bear.

After checking for possible injuries, I frantically thought back to what the hospice nurse had said to do in the event of a fall: rely on a surface such as a nearby bed. (There was none.) Tie a belt around his waist to aid in any lifting. I grabbed one, wrapped it around his waist, and tried to hoist him a mere few inches. No success. Swallowing panic, and noting the darkness of night outside, my words, "Shall I call a neighbor? Maybe Helen's husband?" brought a brave "We can do it. Just give me time to get my breath."

So we waited.

We tried again, and after a few false starts, I got him up on his knees.

We waited again, and on surveying the area for some low, soft things, I eventually rigged a series of firm pillows that led up to a low chair onto which I was able to tug him.

The physical effort nearly killed me. Though I had managed to engineer the feat, I had almost passed out from the exertion.

The incident scared us both, and my inner voice screamed, never again.

THINGS I CAN DO

Because I am feeling so helpless these days, I struggle to identify specific ways I can actually help David:

Pretend that the sun is shining.
Cry silently in the sink while the potatoes boil.
Pray.
Order Chinese take out.
Take him for a ride.
Kiss his balding head.
Update both our calendars.
Ignore the national politics.
Remember the wedge of cheese for his apple pie.
Just be there, near and beside him.

BOXES

David's thirty-one boxes of loose memorabilia stored in our basement cease to be a laughing matter. Procrastination rears its ugly head, so I threaten to back up the pickup to the basement door and transport the assortment to the local Durham dump. "Would it make any difference if I sprinkled dollar bills throughout?" he mischievously asks?

Gradually, one by one, I carry the boxes up from the basement to accompany our winter evenings. He thoughtfully sorts the letters and photos stamped the year '54, '73, '89. The task becomes pleasurable as the paper mementos become surprising reminders of a life fully lived.

"I bet Larry would enjoy this old photo."

"My sister will get a kick out of this."

So he starts sending the treasures back to their sources. He passes on the pleasure of the forgotten: evidence he had bailed a friend out of jail brings a smile to his comely face, and a thank you from parents for loaned money brings the response "did I do that?" Soon the exercise stimulates phone calls of delight. Personal contacts are heartedly resumed.

And would Ripley believe that a lifetime guarantee on binoculars once purchased in Germany brings a free repair in 2002?

CHRISTMAS AGAIN

From the warmth of our sitting room we watch the colorful blinking lights on our neighbor's indoor tree. Our fifth Christmas with illness center stage.

I invite all the relatives to celebrate here on Christmas day and on December 28th, the usual trip to Hanover no longer possible for David. There is much preparation to be done, and close friends are aghast that entertaining is on my menu, but the anticipated laughter and children's antics blot out the fact that this will be our last holiday together.

An unexpected snowstorm adds to the scene on Christmas day. After the excitement of opening presents from Santa, but before romping outside, the young and old dip into David's collection of prehistoric warm long underwear. Garbed in the museum quality winter apparel—heavy wool Johnson pants, red hunting outfits, and Chinese fur hats—they bring laughter and tears to those peering out. Jayne, age six, wants a snowman. Leah struggles into oversize boots, and Kayley defends herself against her brothers' snowballs.

The Swenson dinner party on December 28th brings Iwonka's surprise visit, a rifle's passage from one generation to another, and a digital portrait by the fireplace. Too big a crowd for the dining room, we spread ourselves around what the realtor has called an "elegant farmhouse," balancing China plates on our knees, making merry random talk.

I direct my thoughts to David—you sit as comfortable as possible on your folding wheelchair seat and watch your loved ones. I know that any talking now an effort, but few note that you seldom speak. Just being together is your treasured gift of these December moments.

MUSIC

It is Sunday.

Listening to the car radio while returning from a rush trip to the local market, I am suddenly mesmerized by the sweetness of a male tenor. Who is it? What is the music? A fifth-century mass?

I reach home but remain sitting in the car, stupefied by the purity of tone, the crystalline beauty and simplicity of the music.

I wait for the credits to be announced and the station name to be repeated. I note the time, and, after turning off the engine and unloading the groceries in the kitchen, I hastily prepare to make a call of inquiry.

Later that day I learn that at the exact moment of feeling electrified by the exquisite Monteverdi music, our very good friend Alan, an Episcopal priest, had a massive heart attack in the pulpit, dying soon thereafter.

Stunned, David and I both acknowledge not only what Alan had meant to us back at St. Paul's, but at the powerful invisible connection that music has always been, and will continue to be, as a central part of the love in our lives.

DESKS

Across the hall David sleeps more and more.

Today I commence war games with my desk.

Before beginning the packing, I must attack the bills and all that unopened junk mail that threatens to make orderly boxing impossible: somebody's annual report, a new Medicare directory, pleas for money, new e-mail addresses, political declarations, weird unsolicited catalogs, notifications of disconnections, magazine coupons, a survey about nursing home preferences, a police benefit.

If I stop to read everything I won't have time to prepare David's favorite supper. I make hasty decisions, meaning, I separate the bills and toss the problems into the circular file. Eating a stray brownie moves me along.

Too bad I'm not one of those organized zealots.

MOVING II

I sort, discard, give away, donate, sell, tear up, file.

Dismantling a house in a hurry is impossible. A three-story 150-year-old farm-house with endless corners and collected clutter reduced to manageable boxes? Beat the clock?

I grew up on hymns like "We Would Be Building" sung to the mighty tune of *Finlandia*. From rector sets, blocks, and Lincoln logs, I saw myself give one pebble at a time to the creation of something, like a fragile second grader's gift for Mom, a school project, that invisible goal. For others, it may become an architectural skyscraper wonder.

I once saw the fragility of what could go wrong when a modest hut was built on the tide line in the evening by a youth group. Morning brought stark truths about the effort of formation and how outside forces can relentlessly break down and destroy the best of intentions.

Why doesn't someone teach us the best way to deal with dismantling?

Total letting go is torture.

Reduction is more than price.

MOVING III

I conclude that the chaos of moving would be too stressful for David, so plans to place him under hospice/hospital care for three days are in order. A social worker lines up the Care-Van transportation and starts the admittance procedure of necessary paperwork. We both endure an anxious preparation time for the separation.

I follow the van and discover on arrival that physical exhaustion has suddenly hit me. Too weak to tote his small suitcase to the single room at the hospital, I momentarily collapse and seek aid.

Friday morning back at home, the day before the movers arrive, I survey the disheveled mess of pre-moving day. My daughter Laurie, mother of five, arrives from Massachusetts, checks my list of things to do, and efficiently starts taking down curtains and doing the kitchen packing. A friend Suzanne works on the refrigerator and delivers Amos the cat to friend Shirley. Dick and Ben carefully pad and take away artwork. Anne drops off a yummy cake for tomorrow's workers; Helen drops by and insists on dinner at her expense; Norma fills her trunk with the last sacks of book donations; and I fall onto the stair chair for the very last time. I glide upwards, without my merry song, to attack the screaming-to-be-done upstairs bedrooms.

MOVING IV

We move between snowstorms. The day is fodder for a slapstick movie.

The truck gets stuck twice in our long driveway, once requiring a call to AAA for assistance, once blocking traffic on busy Route 4. The loading is barely finished by dusk, so, the promised same-day unloading is postponed until Monday.

But church friends appear and are fantastic! The afternoon troops include: two couples who make dump runs after traipsing up and down the narrow old back stairway with sacks of old *Stone Digest* magazines; a buyer for the drafting table; Concord friend Pat, who carts plants and breakables to the condo in her own vehicle; two of David's friends, Ben and Dick, who load our woodpile onto our blue truck (in New Hampshire firewood equals cash) and my gracious hired cleaning crew, who work into the night.

Ben gets the contents of the liquor cabinet, and a mover employee gets David's office couch.

MOVING V

Sunday Carolyn and I visit David at the hospital. It is his birthday, so we take a cake. Although we're anxious to share humorous details of the weekend fiasco, we are glad to see him looking rested and refreshed. The room feels strangely sterile, metallic, and neat.

Together we remember his birthday of last year—a shared celebration for twelve in a private Durham dining room at an elegant country inn in Durham. He is part of a unique group of February birthday babies who, over the years, had often enjoyed sitting down together in the seclusion of their homes to share ludicrous greeting cards and playful gifts. Warmed by fond memories, we especially recall many of those gatherings around the fireplace and piano at Bert Whittemore's family "estate."

But I see fear in David's eyes.

He does not like it here in the hospital. Is he fearing abandonment? So it is especially good when David's brother Malcolm and family from Hanover arrive. And phoned birthday greetings give Carolyn and I a chance to slip away to sleep on the condo floor before getting to unpack the same tired stuff the very next day.

PERMANENCE

Whatever happened to "pencil it in?"

Sitting by David's new bed as he dozes, I find myself doing Cryptogram puzzles in ink. I do not know why I choose this kind of puzzle or why I am preferring to use a pen. Erasing is messy? Can't find a pencil? Ink forces me to be careful from the beginning?

None of the above; I need to feel that something is definite.

In the back of my mind float thoughts like find an electric razor for him, remember Rick's birthday, be home when the commode will be dropped off. Forget the shock of discovering that the washer and dryer were not included in the sale or that the new sleeper couch didn't fit through the entry door.

It is hard to deal with the temporary in everything, with the feelings of no set tomorrows. Or I might never get to a final rendition. The now is all I have, and it is like relearning life to stay in the moment. It requires a different kind of discipline that ignores the possibility of change as a normal part of living.

Was temporary once okay? Is haste now always disastrous? What is today's motto? Is it permanent?

We listen to Josh Groban's line "You are Mine Forever."

We pin it down so it doesn't slip away.

TRUCK

David privately tells Steven he wants him to have his blue truck. Steve is incredulous, and broadcasts this to each of us over and over again during those last weeks. In whispers of reverence, the paperwork is discussed by phone and duly carried out.

The big day comes; it is the week before David's death.

His father, Rick, drives Steve up from Massachusetts. The essential keys somehow change hands.

David and I watch from the condo window as Steve turns to wave. Tears well up as we watch the simultaneous emotions of love for a grandfather and the joy of being the recipient of the big Dodge widebody that will become his proud transportation for commuting to college.

Another wave, another thanks again, seals David's pleasure in the exchange as he himself turns back to the bedroom, weary. To use a nice old New England analogy, he then drops down "like a Stoughton bottle."

HUMILITY

It is a joy to watch friends express their love to David. One can almost see the momentary shift from stagnant self to a flowering conscious-ness of the other. The reach is spontaneous yet generous and gentle, portraying a basic inner sanctity so often withheld.

There seems to be a subtle preparation of self to be in the pres-ence of the dying—a braveness, a self brought forward, a keenness, a conscious decision to see and appreciate the pure, the best.

We all are camouflaged, dulled by labor, tedious repetitions, meaningless activity, discouragement, but also capable of letting go of the burden of a disguised, unwieldy self.

The sick person's part in the dialogue of death is real, as evidenced in the stark honesty of the young man at a funeral who voiced his first-time anxiety on visiting a cancer-ridden friend. He had been deeply touched by the way *she* welcomed him. Just as always, joyfully, internally unchanged.

Why are we expected to be different when we're dying?

SAYING GOOD-BYE

What is the language of parting? How do we proofread the willingness, the timing, the letting go? Can we reword the usual concept of last days so that those lingering on can go forth, fully living day by day, feeling still valued, even rejoicing?

Other deaths have been endured. Death has already been preceded by other endings, such as summer camp drop-offs, wartime separations, knocks on the door in the night, catastrophic events that allowed no time for kissing farewells.

If we are participating in someone's dying, might we not be privileged to acknowledge that the future for them could be filled with light? Death but a passing to a better place, part of the normal sequence of a round of healthy living?

If we're lucky, our faith clicks in, our farewells get spoken, and our God grips us firmly as readable human signs of affection are topped off by the mysterious and the everlasting.

LAST DAYS

I am in a logjam. The condo is cramped and crowded.

The hospice nurse has explained that the end is near, the expected six months rudely shortened. David has slept in the sunny corner bedroom for less than two weeks.

Special friends stop by, making their own last good-byes. Charlie changes the fire alarm battery. Dick adjusts the new-to-me kind of furnace thermostat, my sister and niece bring food, Betty chats with the living room drop-ins, Carolyn sings an aria for David, tears streaming.

Everything accelerates. There are demands. It's a frenzy. There is no privacy.

Which way do I turn? What is left of time outrages me! My beloved is slipping away in this terrible sweep of drama, all erratically paced amidst raw kindness and speeded-up momentum.

Stop! Stop!

Leave David and me alone!

Let us die together!

Instead, I carefully measure out his liquid relief into a common-place weathered kitchen spoon.

COMA

David is now in a semi-coma.

My beautiful husband, his regal face, his once loving arms, so still.

The hospice nurse provides lollipop gadgets to moisten his mouth. They look like pieces of pink spun candy on a stick and are meant to bring relief to a very dry mouth. Kneeling by the bed, I soak in these last precious hours, loving him, keeping him close, for that unknown number of minutes and heart-rending hours.

Steve leaves school on the south shore and rushes to David's bedside. His "It's me, Grandpa, Steven" brings the last, single flicker of eye contact.

Carolyn and I watch him constantly for signs of bodily discomfort. He appears to be sleeping soundly now. Aware that patients in a coma may be able to hear, Carolyn sings one of his favorites softly.

I am still haunted by my first husband's need for chopped ice for his dry mouth and a wave of anger surfaces within my desperate words: "Are those little swabs considered a sign of progress in our great big bragged-about medical world?" Just dunk them, I'm told, not only in water but a little light fruit juice.

Such small stabs at making him whole and happy and awake and mine again.

195

CIRCLES OF LOVE

We form a circle around the bed—my grandson Ian, Carolyn, Reverend Pirie, and myself.

We hold hands to fight back the demon of death, to try to hold him a few more minutes in the loving forces of our protective thoughts, but at the same time letting him go, launching him, into what has to be a better place, a place of peace and justice and relief. "Thank God he doesn't have to struggle to breathe anymore," says his faithful friend Ben at a later date.

Led in prayer, heads bowed, we commit him, releasing him to a power far beyond ourselves, drawing on a ritual practice from ages past, feeling strength and sweetness invade the room, encompassing his blessed body and soul.

The community of faith solemnly sending forth.

It is Valentine's Day.

GONE

I am a damaged lobster trap
I am a shuttered window
I am day-old bread
My husband is gone, and I too am a missing person.

Bereft of his tenderness
I cannot cry
I cannot even talk to myself.
But then

I see him polishing his shoes
I see him savoring his shredded wheat
His face is on the pillow beside me
He is not really gone.

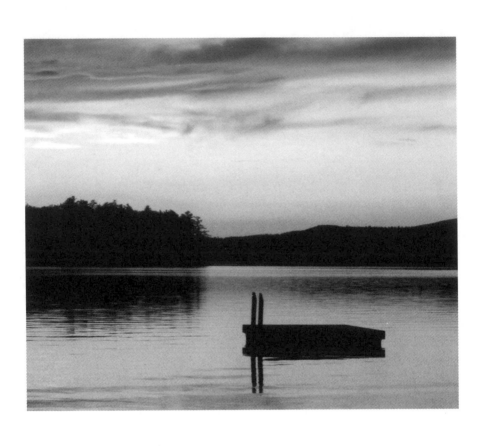

THE AFTERTHOUGHTS

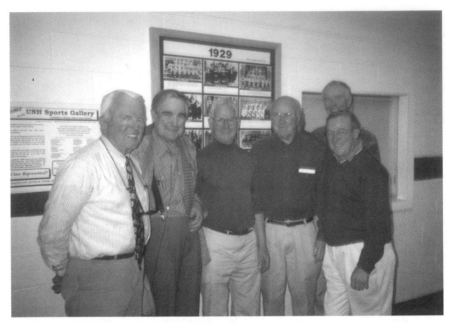

Concord friends.

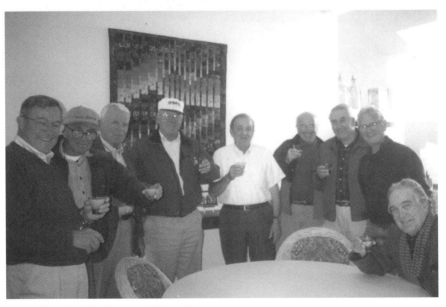

Last days with Concord friends.

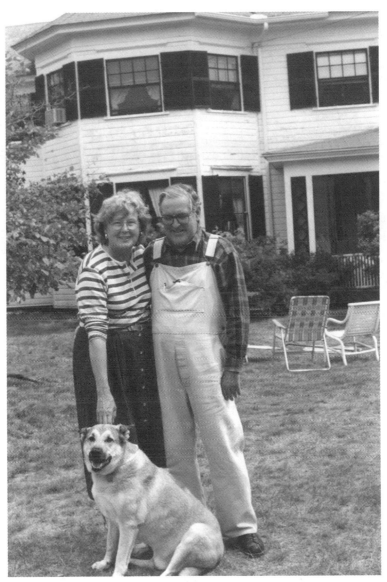

Cecil and David's favorite overalls.

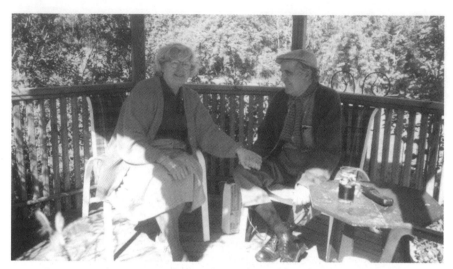

Together in Durham Gazebo.

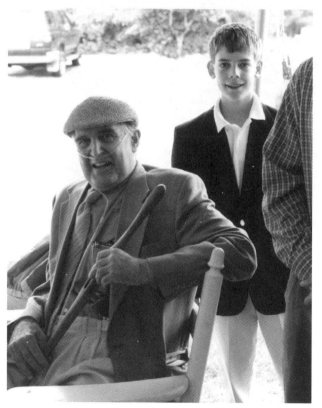

The two Davids.

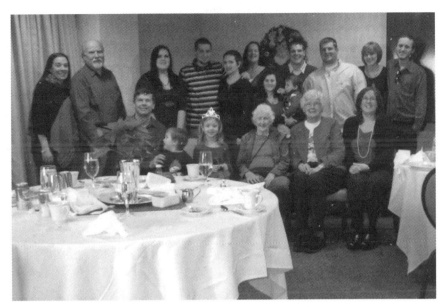

Hotel Christmas; the Sheraton.

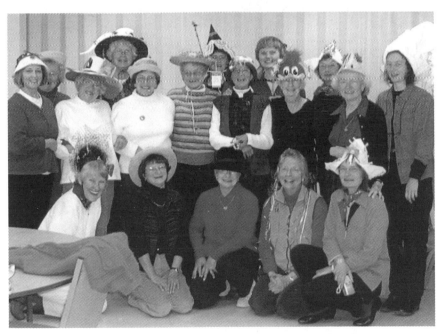

Harriet leads conference on aging.

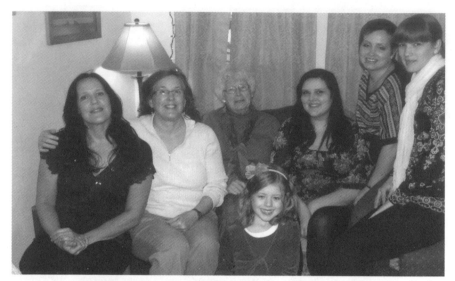

The Clark girls on vacation in York, Maine.

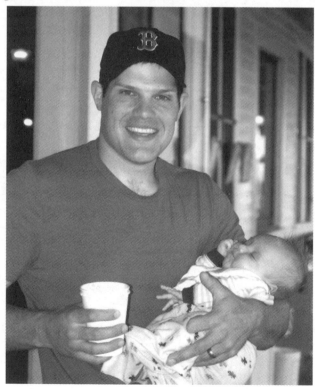

A new great grandson, Owen, with his father Steve.

VI. Without

ornings are silent now.

M The cat sits by the glass deck door glancing out, saying
nothing.

The dying does not go away; it advances. In spite of the six years
of knowing, I am not ready.

Carolyn and I together try to draft an obituary. Slumped at the
dining room table with blank white paper, we strain to jot down
notable facts that might define the story of an exceptional man.
When we insert statements like "incredible ability to make and maintain friendships" the *Concord Monitor* editor tells us "they" use only
formula writing, to which "we" of course rebel in good old New
England fashion. Three drafts later, the personal touches intact, we
bullishly wend it off to acceptance and plenty of positive comments.

I feel like an invalid and want only to hunker down on my
favorite wing back chair, out of sight, and read lengthy novels to
gobble up time.

Our two clergy, with a sizable funeral now on their agenda,
solemnly visit as I sit numb and wordless. Choose a date, the soloist,
the order of service, a favorite hymn. All I can manage to contribute
is the selection of a hymn, *"When Love is Found"* before my brain
mercifully shuts down. Explicit plans fail to knife through the blur
of gouged-out emptiness. Thank God David had chosen the funeral
home in advance.

In spite of blizzard conditions, many friends and relatives did flock to Dover First Parish Church, though I recall little more than rushed trips to the bathroom, which confused dear Steven, my gallant chauffeur for the day. I just sit numbly in a pew between my two lovely daughters (closed airports keep my son in DC.)

I pretend I am present but I am not. Almost senseless, I am aware only of the large symbolic granite blocks provided for the altar by cousin Kevin. Words from the precious Psalms are read, as were faxes from associates worldwide, DC relatives and town dump personnel, witnessing one last time David's rare portrayal of the word "integrity." With feet burning from standing in an endless receiving line, I accept my kind son-in-law's invitation to dinner at the spacious UNH New England Center Restaurant. Amidst the hushed feasting, I silently find myself harboring that crazy fabled wish—that a loon might be heard accompanying dear David to a beauteous afterlife somewhere.

Then the weeks drag by.

With outside circumstances ceasing to dictate my life, I find I am still caught in a fog of nothingness:

What comes next?

Who needs me?

Who cares?

Who am I now?

Even the psalmist cried out a plea of "help me," "hear me," "why has thou forgotten me?"

As the days crawl by, nothing seems important. I can't remember what I like to eat, yet I'm not really hungry and make do with chips and Chinese takeout. Why eat, anyway? There's only me! Or I lock the car door and leave the window open.

My body aches, yet sleep eludes me. Years of staying up with David till the last midnight medicines are taken have left me in a debilitated state.

Do I want to take a walk? Should I unpack another box? Six green gumdrops could do the trick. Someone says when in doubt, do the laundry.

Alone in the condo those early weeks, I felt like the old lady who muttered: "Sometimes I sit and think. Sometimes I just set."

I decide that grief is like a dusting of new snow, touching every leaf and shrub of my earthbound afterlife. It is thorough. It does not let me escape. The wind of life could blow the powder away, or, if the sun should break through, it could spread minute diamond sparkles that etch minuscule patterns into my withering perspective, allowing a gradual thawing. I mean hope, that thing with feathers, according to a poet. Or hope, furtively referenced by Garrison Keillor's comic "Hopeful Gospel Quartet." Hope is not a choice but a moral obligation, according to someone else. Yes, a phantasmal coverlet that hovers and floats with snippets of peace and acceptance appearing if the sun can eventually puncture my cold, frosted, blue, lingering doubts.

The next day I decide that grief is like a large fishing net thrown across oceanic waters. I again see the long-ago sight at Star Island of a mighty commercial vessel with its giant mechanical arm pitching out a hundred-foot net from a high tower. The net is a slick design that brutally captures a whole school of unsuspecting fish innocently darting to and fro in the freezing turquoise depths below. I feel tackled, like those swarming fish, wrestling with grisly forces to survive. My steady twinkly-eyed lover has left me to fend for myself in the bottomless cold waters of human life. Caught and hooked. Doomed and pushed back into the mainstream. Back where I know that giving David's widow the once-over would be part of the inevitable, unavoidable game plan.

I'm probably depressed.

Then again, there was that supernatural time at dusk, during a light falling snow, when I sensed movement beyond my sliding glass door. About to view MacNeil and his six o'clock news as I lay back in my wicker rocker that had once graced the Lynnfield church nursery, I managed to idly glance outside and count eight deer silently feeding in the wooded area by our small pond. It felt like a sign. For one precious moment I was mesmerized, infused with the wonder of life and the delicacy of living things. While probably feeling totally isolated, those lovely four-footed creatures formed a subtle message from the outer limits that God's natural beauty and caring will not desert me—if I am alert and open to the awareness of the divine in everything, even in pain.

It surprises me that I am remembered.

Letters and notes of condolence pour in. So many kind people take time to tell me about their love for David and their concern for me. Who said that men can't express their feelings well? And this included a personal call from David's primary care physician, Dr. Decker. And today it's a prayer shawl from a Star Island friend. The minister's wife delivers the pussy willows from David's funeral bouquet. Kurt sends powerful verses from a favorite poet. Bonnie drives up from Weston and feeds me. And I can hear David, on shaking his head, say, "you got a raw deal" which I had bravely denied, but as the immensity of loss sinks in and I thaw out, I scream "what is left for me?" to the shadows of late afternoon descending. I swallow the quip "it must be five o'clock somewhere," and proceed to treat myself to the last drops of David's Smirnoff.

A few weeks later my dreary state is interrupted by the fact that the lease on my car is up. Then I become a stranger, a disjointed, rebellious dance performer being dragged onto a macadam dance floor of polished models and sickening sticker prices. Just looking I say. My survey tells me what I do not want to know. A slow waltz onto a second lot confirms there will be no dates with bargains. A friend loans me *Consumer Reports*, and my daughter puts me through not a foxtrot but a financial pace. If the price is A, the interest rate B, how many months of payments will pay off the cursed indebtedness? She makes a cute little chart and watches me dicker and twist.

The search for a used low-mileage deal being what all widows want, we form a square dance of strangers shifting forward and back. I do a ghost dance around a Subaru whose interior reeks of smoke. I grimace, then bravely refrain from brawl-like action with another saucy but smirking salesman. Eventually I say good-bye to my leased and merry leather-seated Oldsmobile, and climb up into my spiffy green second-hand Honda CRV. Whew. That shindig is over.

The next month I get lucky.

Ian, my oldest grandson, leaves his college class early and drives to New Hampshire to spend time with me. Of course, the condo is still a disaster area of unpacked boxes, necessities, and minimal food-stuffs in wrong places, but as he is the family computer whiz he goes right to work assembling my computer ensemble, after which we go out to lunch and I get to stand proudly beside his stocky football build. It's such a relief that the grandchildren still come—over the river and through the woods to a cold condo and a desolate Grandma instead of a large cozy farmhouse with window boxes, high-ceilinged guest bedrooms, and a one-of-a-kind grandfather. The ups and downs of medical conditions are gone, but some things remain. When I open the refrigerator, it still offers me alien contents, but I am inventing new games of grocery survival. I may start with buying one peach, one banana, and one tomato so there will be cash left for two pieces of chocolate.

Ben, David's friend from Phillips Andover days, calls periodically to "see how you're doin." He's one of the only ones with whom I feel I can openly declare "I miss him so!" He doesn't fear that I'm falling apart or will embarrass him or will sob uncontrollably. He doesn't cover up feelings with jokes because Ben knows better; his wife had been an invalid for many years. When he responds quite simply with "I know you miss him" he really means it. And he brings out a picture taken a few weeks before that fatal Valentine's Day of David's death. David with his swollen face is surrounded by five of his faithful friends, I think how lucky he was!

What upsets me most is coming across the scribbled list of final household jobs that had to be completed on that last moving day. "I've got a little list!" I told Gilbert who still taunts me about it. Who could have been in charge of that? I gasp. Roll up office rugs, take down living room curtains, fix door to the linen closet, get the slate welcome sign off the front porch. Orders and deadlines, as in military instructions. Do I know who that frantically efficient, organized, speedy person was? Me? I almost vomit. Four columns of jobs to be done according to son-in-law, grandson, a daughter, and myself. Details atop the stress and care of my husband. Who was this person? Certainly not someone like myself who prefers silent reflection and backdoor participation. A new identity problem?

Someone please praise me. Then again, maybe the self we think we are doesn't exist. Or grief is making me into someone else. I'm not a wife or a lover now but an increasingly frugal, organized sergeant. I only know I miss him, and still wear his navy plaid nightshirt to bed. I am trapped in yardage of empty times, all in sharp contrast to my former role of monitoring doctor appointments, and clocking visitors, interruptions, and departures.

I crave that special dose of kindness that only a loving mate can provide.

Even the cat is having a hard time making adjustments. I miss Amos' midnight moans of the feline hunting ritual as he chases the mice that once peppered our Williams Way address. Now, on only occasional evenings, he becomes a wild mountain goat, scampering over the abridged complement of furniture, streaking through the small rooms in wild exasperation

I know a cat doesn't kiss or bark, but later his comforting bundle of warm self in my lap each evening creates a temporary bond. It suffices.

Eventually, I venture out. Out from my cocoon of private, safe, familiar readables to a strange new world dominated by groupings: husbands and wives together, young lovers touching, kids in clubs and teams in batches, laughing and clowning. I just move in short spurts. The simplest of self-care duties requires Herculean effort: I took a shower today. Hallelujah. Yesterday I took out the big white garbage bag. Hooray.

Shopping becomes a new kind of disease. Where else can you wander about, in slow motion, without speaking, crying incognito at the sight of that familiar shirt or get a little exercise without changing into your sweats? What is on display behind glass windows does not demand anything from me. I can observe and glide on to view the same merchandise in a different store, but I don't have to buy it. "It doesn't matter, matter, matter."

I move furniture around the condo and add lilac wallpaper to one bedroom wall.

I try a few simple exercises. I cannot imagine returning to the rigorous Tai Chi class, so I try mindfulness. Sit quietly, concentrate on breathing in and out while thinking love in, peace out. It does help, but it is often the sight of a cardinal or a mallard that tips my scale of precarious balance.

I can now go back to enjoying blocks of time to touch, feel, and concentrate on making another quilt. When friend Pat sees my jumble of bright psychedelic colors against "black backgrounds" lying on my quilting table, she screams, "Those are mine! My favorites!" So I decide I will make this one for her, the dark stashes of deep color chosen hastily during David's illness. It is an opportunity to bring pleasure to my friend by way of miniature birds in a variation of the Irish Chain pattern. I delve into making something of beauty that will bring pleasure to another. As I had once designed and marketed fabricated wall hangings for corporate space—partly based on my belief that I was brightening up the lives of those caught in nine to five boredom—I would return to a one to one gift. In the process of some silent sewing, David comes back to me. How do I know? Because a Great Blue Heron does his three-point-landing, without warning, into the small pond out back. I know he is there before I see him. Of course, to me, David has never left. His sweet presence is a permanent part of my life as I struggle to go on living. Like the great bird, David is my silent partner.

> "I long for the sound
> of your voice.
> The face
> I see so clearly
> Doesn't say a word"
>   —Japanese poet

But the fact that a winter death automatically postpones burial in New England until spring or summer is a bummer. Having barely crawled an iota out of the numbness of loss, I must step back into it again and be responsible, act strong. It is like swimming upstream. Certain feelings about the graveside service can now flow forth, and

I am thankful it gives me a chance to express my grief, unlike at the funeral, where I was numb to anything offered.

So ideas simmer that June. My love of literature enables me to get to the heart of love and grief and loss and gratitude. I search through many texts and decide on a series to be read by three voices: Barbara, my sister-in-law, Reverend Jed Reardin, a favorite UCC pastor in Concord where the burial will be held, and my own.

To honor David's dog Cecil, I first paraphrase Matthew Fox's famous canine tribute, and include a letter by David about his own frugal childhood, lines from poet May Sarton, and of course W. H. Auden's "He was my North, my South, my East, my West." Then I send each attendee home with an Elliott Rose, and David's brother Malcolm provides a family picnic on the granite company lot nearby where all agree that David would have wholeheartedly approved both the ambiance and the frugality.

The following day I return to Concord to stand at his grave. I crave to be alone with him as Carolyn's exquisite "Pie Jesu" from the Fauré Requiem over the open grave still lifts my heart to the searing sense of finality that a burial becomes. After the anguish of long-term dying, the dreadful moving, the endless winter, I yearned to tell him things he might want to know, all while envisioning his loving blue eyes upon me, so filled with his own distinct way of expressing our magnetic connection.

The spacious hillside cemetery was alive with spring flowering shrubs, winding walkways, fluttering military markers, and an occasional jogger passing silently through. I at last felt calmed but emptied, honored, blessed, and grateful for the exceptional variety of color and design in headstones proud witnesses to the many granite quarries that once graced this area. To be alone with my beloved served a desperate need. The lushness of greenery seemed to enclose and protect me.

And the tears came. Finally. By the bucket.

In the periodic brooding about the idea of death, I had somehow concluded that death was not the worst culprit. I had survived the last trimester of watching his dying and found I was now thirsting for truth about this natural process.

I believe the birthing process of pushing the baby out needs to be profoundly followed by a reevaluation of letting life go. In a world where facts about birth, abortions, pregnancy, and prenatal care are broadcast out loud, advertised, illustrated, and frankly detailed, I need to know more about death as a good and natural thing, perhaps promising some kind of afterlife. We have been barraged by phrases that use the body as a measuring stick, from "knee-high" to "arm-length." I yearn now to know more about the weights and measures of spirit.

I am straining to see death as the giving back to God, and I have at times been nurtured by the spirit as well as by the body of a person.. That is what lingers on for those of us mourning and remaining. In blunt truth I had worried most about David being free from pain, not the actual act of dying. When death came, I wept most from disbelief, exhaustion, and relief.

With spring came a nudge to breathe fresh air and eventually do the garden thing. There is no helpful fellow in faded coveralls pushing a worn brown wheelbarrow in my direction, no wooden sawhorse holding handsome planters waiting to be painted. There is only me. Two days later, I grab a small bag of potting soil at Agway; and three days later a cheap blue child's garden tool at Zyla's discount. I tell myself I will plant it on Saturday at ten o'clock. There might be a place by the lower-level door. So I do the deed silently —gritting my teeth, getting it over with, and all the while see his hands doing the gentle setting, the moderate watering; his strong hands securing the young plantings into their fragile new places in the merciful sun.

Gardens. A continuing. A small sign of life, a gesture, a tribute, my first whack at doing it again.

Actually, what I am doing is allowing myself to be consoled by the natural world. Or sometimes I read ferociously and survive weekends accompanied by *Book TV*. In July I walk on Jenness Beach alone, immersing myself in summertime memories of sunny times there at the beach with him.

We had often joined the grandchildren in riding the modest waves, on small white foam boards. And I can still see the look of pleasure on David's tanned face after his hastily caught ride, with the stumbling up the beach and the yanking up of his red polyester bathing trunks. Then we would turn and do it again and again, joyfully catching the salty waves, inhaling the sound of the surf unfolding on the whitewashed sand, one of the miraculous things that stays the same.

Mail is still coming addressed to David saying he's prequalified for a new Visa card with zero percent financing.

Anticipation of our "magic place" in September keeps me going through the rest of the summer. That and the vision of his courage and determination as I return to some regular church attendance, I remember him climbing the church's steep exterior granite stairs, fresh, clean, and neat in his camel jacket, white shirt, and colorful tie. He would climb slowly, then stop and rest. Lean to the left on the wrought iron railing while grasping the strap of his portable oxygen tank in his right. One. Two. Three. Others seldom understood. A few politely waited, a few nodded to his pleasant greeting, and some told him to take the side entrance, for Pete's sake, not understanding his challenging self-setting goal.

Then in August, with fear and trembling, I return to the annual Star Island Conference with the children. Pack my things to go to a place where the ocean water is frigid, cold showers are rationed, and I will helplessly remember when both of my husbands once mingled there, with me and a million squawking seagulls. I sleep in cottage C or prop myself in a porch rocker to stare at lively children, the quaint harbor, and the nearby tennis matches. I play latenight bridge, sing in the historic chapel, and most excitedly dare to take on a new skill with a professional teacher: African drumming. It magically draws me, trancelike, into another almost hypnotic sphere of meaning. I can't help remembering that after the death of my first husband in 1975, I had been invited to speak there in the chapel on what it's really like to be a widow in our culture. What a powerful response there had been, as the subject at that time was taboo.

Come September, David's absence at the lake is so painful I can hardly breathe.

He is at the table by the picture window. He is on the porch, smiling over his carefully measured martini, his fist full of peanuts. We are laughing together over Bill Bryson's humorous commentary on America. Fortunately, I had decided to invite my sister and single daughter to each spend a few days there with me, and their cheerful efforts kept me sane. But the days alone bring the great emptiness to the surface. He who had been the center of all that I was would never again grace my life. I ignore the dishes and concentrate on the sunset, meditate, swim each day (swimming off the wide open shoreline restores my spirit), and talk to my wild ducks. Then I quilt and read and learn to slumber there without him, relaxing into the torturous truth of his absence.

A lot has been said about the despair of the first Christmas alone. Well, I just dodge the queries of "what are your plans?" To say I don't have any disturbs those with fixed traditions. What I mean is, I don't want to plan things without him. His attitude about holidays had always been relaxed. Now mine is, too. Thank you, David, for teaching me that real giving is not by company policy, family expectation, or cultural orders, but spontaneously from the heart. Of course we ladies still get out our holiday earrings and Santa Claus sweaters and do a great job of ignoring the eggnog or mistletoe rituals.

Now, there are no boxes to lug down from the attic.

There is no attic.

But I do get out the ancient crèche bought the year that young Bill was born, and the damaged cow and the chipped blue shepherd remind me of the blessed journey I have been able to make.

February means his birthday, our anniversary, and his death, with the approach of Valentine's Day sending me into a spin. I do the kind of pretending that exhausts me.

The memory of our wedding at St. Paul's Church and then our reception at the Society for the Protection of New Hampshire Forests is etched on my soul forever.

When I retrieve a video of Concord, New Hampshire and view my beloved being interviewed about granite's history, I expect to weep at the sight and sound of his living presence. Instead, I am shocked by his already swollen face, years before his actual death. But February 14 brings warm expressions of love, including a long walk on the beach with friend Pat, and the delivery of fresh new kindling from cousin Tom.

So I hang in there and hug any sunshine that is offered.

My first year without him.

VII. Living with Grief

I slowly saunter back into the mainstream while new habits and rhythms begin to emerge. I try to reconcile brushfires of energy and the bundles of apathy that dictate my days. I don't cry from joy anymore when I see a Vermeer painting, but I weep after Hurricane Irene on seeing a rescue dog on TV save a helpless dog.

My first stab at so-called "work" since David's death is a workshop. A friend, Ellen, has asked me to design one for her. She wants to invite a large group of favorite women over a certain age to Geneva Point Retreat Center on Lake Winnipesaukee, New Hampshire, for a weekend so they can impart wisdom directly to her as she prepares for her sixtieth birthday. She knows I have led retreats on aging for churches, and created spiritually oriented programs for seniors at the Pine Mountain Conference Center.

She makes suggestions of what we could include, and her positive attitude lifts me out of feelings of isolation to consider taking it on. We agree on the focus of "celebratory," and settle down to review effective ways of sharing life experiences.

It is a rousing success! Through some small group work, a lot of laughter, percussion instruments loaned from a UNH group, Pat's uplifting worship, and the invention of our very own rituals of late adulthood, what began as a gathering of strangers became a landmark event for my friend and a force toward healing for me.

Yes, I would like more laughter in my life, and yes, I want things like a new dump sticker. I would like to have a geography lesson, too. I cannot find Yugoslavia, and Burma has disappeared. Yet do we really know what we really want? We build porches we don't sit on, or design picture windows we cover up. I at least really want my life sprinkled with whiskers and wags. Animals bring to me not only companionship but what an Indian chief once explained: "if the beast were gone, we would die from a great loneliness of spirit." At the same time I'm supposed to be worrying about credit card fraud and identity theft. Now I ask you, does the "what will I wear today" still outdo the "how can I contribute justice and compassion and peace?"

Painfully, I am slowly moving David's clothing along, but I cannot move it all out. I like each article's continuing reference point. So it's suspenders to Andy, a warm woolen jacket to my brother, and an opportunity for the grandsons Ian and Steve to choose something to treasure. I sort a few of David's things at a time, finger the heavy ski socks or the Andover cap, but my favorite sweater of his will probably hang in my closet forever. If I hurriedly pass it along, would I then be able to bear it?

I deliver certain useful items, such as the raised toilet seat, the maroon walker, and the shower chair, to others who have similar needs.

The longer Amos the cat and I share this small condo, the more we become alike. I think I am adopting animal instincts. For example, I am now able to spot a movement in the brush out back that might be a bear or a moose. But I do not have a tail to swish, and easily forget the confinements of the twenty-four hour day.

Amos, in turn, is exhibiting human reactions. Expecting dinner at five, he lolls on the bed, not the floor, and communicates modest but regular needs for affection. Sometimes we have "conversations." When he rushes to a window, I tend to ask, "is there something I should know?" And I, in turn, am learning to decipher the meaning behind a half-cocked meow.

He is also learning English. When I prepare to leave the house, he now knows the difference between my "I'll be right back," "Just a little while," and "I'm sorry, honey, it's going to be a long time." He sighs, calmly turns, and retreats to his favorite living room chair.

When I call the vet, I've been known to say I'm Amos' mother.

They say husbands and wives can grow to look alike. So guess I'll worry only if I develop whiskers or lap my breakfast, or Amos begins each day by brushing his last tooth with Colgate.

I also feel blessed by my wild four-footed friends who drop in. The possum on the open deck just rattled the bird feeder—a nifty design, that feeder, a gift my daughter had wrestled from someone else during that insane Christmas Yankee Swap exchange. It has tiny perches that automatically close up to the weight of squirrel predators sneaking seeds. (I defy convention by ignoring others' fear of bears.) In the summer it's my great blue heron, lanky and fearless, who is either standing knee-deep fishing for snacks or gradually lifting her amazing feathered gray self to be up and off, in slow motion, bomber style. Or it's the red fox, feeling safe in my presence, daintily but warily stepping out of the tangled brush. Or it's the raccoon with his clever fingers. Or it's the muskrat, my synchronized swimmer in the small pond out back, lugging long, straggly grasses back and forth, steadily focused on nesting. Does he count his laps?

I get angry when I read about folks disturbing the habitat of my winged and four-footed loved ones. After all, we're all searching for sustenance in one way or another. I'll root for your habitat, friend, if you'll continue to root for me.

Sometimes I just talk to David in the welcome sunlight on the deck, and tell him this or that, like the family on Central Avenue finally fixed their fence, and granddaughter Kayley dyed her hair red, and grandson Ian started his own painting business.

Of course I'm still practicing a bit of frugality. I discontinued the *New York Times* when the Sunday price went up. I found a bargain yesterday at Red's Shoe Barn in Dover, to which my family makes the comment, "Why are you wearing basketball sneakers?"

As to handling the finances, right now I'm on overload. Gone are the days of finding milk money pennies for grade-school lunches. It is 2012 and gas is almost four dollars a gallon. When I read that energy prices and food prices are up, I worry. Then the advertising fliers, the utility bills, the sale catalogs pile up in disarray. The premium on my health insurance policy has increased, the church has launched a building campaign and the car payment is due. It is not long before I feel disoriented, floundering in written imperatives, overwhelmed by endless decision making. I brood over more dire messages—Vote NO, Trees Not Towers, yet I remember Gandhi's "my life is my message" and determine to rely on myself.

I revert once in a while to my kind of loneliness. I agree with poet Donald Hall that "this new year is offensive because it will not contain you," but I drive year round with my beach chair in the back of the car. That translates to hope, doesn't it? And I always find time to drive to the Hopkinton area to take lunch to my sister, who now has a serious heart condition, and I regularly visit a bridge friend, Diane, who is battling ALS. Friend Phyllis dies and friend Katherine moves back to Idaho, bringing to mind my daughter Laurie's dreadful childhood exclamation "Everyone dies or moves away!" Then David's brother Andy is diagnosed with cancer, and my son has lost his job. But certain messages of my past are fading. I am learning to tune out meaningless chatter and my mother's "be good, be quiet," my church's "be perfect," my culture's "too old to matter" melts away when my cat's affectionate rubbing posture says "be near me," and I remember David's frequent embrace with its, "I love you, sweetheart."

So, life has a way of moving along. Leah and Adam drive up from Massachusetts and take apart my old computer setup; young Davy goes off to college; and I sew diligently for the church fair. Betty, Malcolm, Andy and lots of Swenson cousins gather each August at a rented coastal property and catch up on our ever-changing lives. We all miss the wonderful summer beach house. The new owners have stripped it down and built a place to make their own kind of memories. Those of us with poignant recollections of its heavily used hallowed spaces still find pleasure in the memories of all those one-of-a-kind gatherings. Now, desperate for a place to be with adult children and grandchildren, I find another roomy old beach house for the children and I to rent in York, Maine, if we all chip in. But I still find myself looking back, wanting to stand still and digest the past.

I find myself mesmerized by some of David's childhood

scrapbooks that his mother had saved. I like to picture him as an earnest young boy, using his eighth grade skills to do the multicolored hand-drawn maps of South America, the black and white sketch of different cloud formations, and the Lady of the Lake study (with an A plus grade). He had an amazing ability to do cartoons, which carried over to his later Yale days. His love of maps is so apparent here, heralding his eventual love of his U.S. Geological Survey collection, which traveled with us in the backseat for so many of our romantic backwoods journeys.

Because of my squirreling habit of tucking away memorabilia, I can also still savor the beauty and romance of various Valentine and Christmas cards from David over the years with words like "I'm so glad I married you," and "to my traveling companion, my lover, my wife." Many of the cards were hand done and designed. "For the woman I love" can stay in my heart for days. "Thank you for marrying me," in David's handsome script, is what truly resonates as I move on to mundane things like the dentist appointment.

When I rummage in another unpacked box of old papers, and see that after the death of my first husband I had paid $450 in property taxes for a large house and yard complete with oceans of lilacs. I now pay $5,500 in taxes for a postage stamp sized condo. I can hear David mutter his favorite commentary of "Good Grief!"

I often sit in the sunny window that I chose for David, but he did not live long enough to enjoy. It is here that pleasurable memories pop back into recollection, and I live again as I relive the sad, the bad, and the remarkable. I had worried so that I would forget "the best." The yesterdays were not forgotten, just buried temporarily. Now the happy and precious occasions often filter to the top and burst forth with joyous remembrance alongside a few tears. I get out the photo albums that bear witness to a variety of unforgettables: the funny beach regalia, the groupings and the graduations, the white water rafting, the Gilbert and Sullivan costuming (David so dashing in his pirate get-up), my Clark family reunions, the fixed smiles, the special occasions. But good memories do prevail (singing around Bert's piano on those shared birthdays), while years of caregiving provide special images such as the dog Cecil's valiant attempt to guard David when strange men had appeared in the bedroom as a response to my 911 midnight call.

I now stop and shop for fabric not because I need a short respite but because that's who I am: a lover of fabric and design and beauty.

The appliance fellow who comes to repair my dryer also fixes my sewing machine. I interpret this not as a regional oddity but a refreshing sign that kindness can spurt forth as easily as a skill deliberately chosen. Has the goodness of people increased?

What is my daily routine now, anyway? I consider. Tuesday afternoons I drop in at the Episcopal Church for the informal gathering of friends for some bridge. I enroll in the new Medicare drug plan, grumbling all the way about another monthly bill. I add a small granite counter to my galley kitchen; when I touch it each day I remember our first tender traipse up Rattlesnake Hill and the thrill of falling in love again.

I volunteer at the Star Island Conference winter office in Portsmouth, New Hampshire. I watch Jeopardy nightly on TV (and get a momentary thrill when Swenson Granite is part of a question about NH) I serve on my condo board, helping to patiently keep track of repairs and headaches of thirty-five units.

Sometimes I'm afraid of Fridays because it can mean watching others rushing to budding affairs while I feel holed up with a cold sandwich and a cat that snores. The cat Amos just got scolded by the vet for weight gain. Lack of exercise, she says. I knew that. He sits a lot, like me, turning old and new thoughts around and around.

I design some women's programs for our church. I know I still need to be bathed in assurance, the adoration of Holy, and some top-level musical expression. Sometimes the pews on Sunday appear to be filled with strangers, but then I see jolly Jean in her wheelchair and Barbara with her sparkling smile. I support the church's thriving new thrift shop. I just sent some of my fabric collection to women of a Zimbabwe church, and I joined our church's new grief support group. But I still bitch about the downtown parking issue. I seem to need a pause that refreshes or a promise sung from a jingling ice cream truck. But instead of complaining I turn it around and connect it to the wine parable, not the Pepsi jingle. I dare to think that maybe I'm now the new product that cannot be contained within outdated concepts.

Of course I still have one of those days—you know—when birds don't sing, the washing machine quits, the printer jams, my credit card disappears.

Amidst the increasing change coming from all directions, I still need David, his kindness, his smarts, his original thinking, his hugs. I still bellow abstract questions, like, "when will I stop saying 'we'?" I still envision my beloved plodder reading his *Book of Common Prayer* each morning at his desk in his den, the nebulizer humming.

Andy Swenson feels better and brings David's siblings together again for a Christmas luncheon in Concord. My son Bill finds a job, and Marie Swenson dies. She was the matriarch who once whispered to me with a mischievous glint in her eyes that David was her favorite Swenson!

When I get serious, I brood about words. Even try humor. When I lose three friends in a week, I say to myself if I'm going to die tomorrow, maybe I should cut my hair or at least clean the bathroom. Words and thoughts can change, be inadequate, or disguise truth and interfere with our understanding of wellness and dying. I fear that we could become more confused and unable to minister to one another. Are there terms that distort your life? Terms like cognitive impairment, eldercare attorney, oncologist, and prednisone. Language is a key to relationships and communication. Do we have a language of caring? What are the words that could lift us up? Words of the heart? Or are we dwelling on all those new words that the medical world is throwing our way?

Reading mysteries continues to be a major diversion. When I read Michael Connelly's opening lines, "death is my beat" I gasp, but I also devour a title like Honorés *In Praise Of Slowness*.

Words from my past come up and haunt me, as in "What shall we do with Grandma?" the opening words to a poem once read to me by a poet I met on the Isles of Shoals. It was a glorious day on the old hotel porch when our minds had idly centered on the expansive view and speculation about aging issues. That had led to the poem about "once you have lived on an island, you will never be the same." Yes, I knew that.

Then, finding meaning in commitment to someone or something, my daughter Carolyn dreams about doing vocal recordings for those experiencing illness, and my niece Elna starts raising money to benefit juvenile diabetes.

I begin to make up my own daily schedule to include dates of outings to artsy events, like viewing sand sculptures at Hampton Beach. I am learning to like going places alone, just as my friend Ethel said I would.

What stays the same? Things like mantras and lyrics, as in "Our God, Our Help in Ages Past." Also being short of cash, and the crazy weather.

I continue to lead my monthly discussion group in exploring aging issues that are otherwise seldom discussed. We have been meeting regularly, nonstop, for twelve years. Our topics of discussion are now richly experiential and have brought us together to a level of intimacy that is very special.

I continue to go to the Isles of Shoals with my family, and when I review the family's commitment and involvement at the Star Island Congregational Conferences, I am thankful that, as a minister's family without roots, we had through the years experienced various roles in a hauntingly beautiful place that became a substitute home: Bill, Sr. a chaplain; Bill, Jr. island historian; Carolyn program chair; Rick and Steven, both youth leaders; Kayley, Laurie and Leah, babysitters.

I still recall the group farewell at the end of the weeklong conference each August on the dock nine miles out at sea with its triple "You Will Come Back," "You Will Come Back," "You Will Come Back" and the shouted triple response by departing conferees on ship "We Will Come Back" is still repeated heartily. (Since 1967 for me, except for the years with illness issues.) It's so wonderful to know there is a healthy, friendly place where the younger generations can experience relational inspiration for our uncertain futures. I learned that living on an island each summer with family had introduced me to tales of pirates as well as a way of living that centers on unconditional love.

I also return to the lake cottage and the loons again a few more times.

Back at home, I like doing David's monthly dump run. I pull in to the transfer station with a happy sense of anticipation, our Durham dump now upgraded. The swap shop has a roof, and the traffic is newly routed. I can line up my Honda SUV behind the red Subaru outback and the Ford pickup truck that is chockfull of UNH student discards, and I wait. I find strange delight in dropping bottles and cans into the great abyss. Tossing is fun. It feels like a cleansing ritual.

David had wanted to know where I would safely be after he died, and though I had assured him I would be all right and not to worry, it is only now that the glow of faith and friends and family on a global scale tell me that life continues to be worth living albeit in new ways and now new places. Whether on stair chair, in memory, or aboard a roller coaster, I am finding my indomitable spirit chugging tentatively on.

I'm really old now, my darling, my rock, my lovable mate.

I no longer color my hair. Bright lights accent the scary wrinkles on the fair skin you once admired. My right leg cramps; things slip out of my arthritic hands. I have degenerated disks in my back, and I just wore a heart monitor for two weeks. I cannot push the vacuum much or walk very far. But I still make lists and the swoop of my Great Blue Heron out back tells me regularly "that all will be well." And now, when I look more closely from my little condo deck, I see there is also a small ugly crane with purple feathers! and what? Orange feet?

"What next, God?" I shout into the landscape, knowing that each of us has felt angry at God at one time or another.

What was next was my sister's death, bringing another period of numbing loss, unleashing those same familiar feelings of helplessness and grief. While born ten years apart, we had had a deep and caring relationship. I miss her. I had lost my brother Walter a few years before, but I still delight in the fact that his last visit from the Maine animal world was a moose who climbed onto his open porch to peek in the window! When Walter "passed," his magnificent oil rendering of a Rembrandt self portrait came to be with me, to grace my tiny condo living room.

I have chain-pieced the sorrow, the treasured moments, the medical madness, the comforting roar of oceans into a one-of-a-kind quilt of a human life. Like others who have been caregivers, I am still on a gradual move—with more scraps, pre-cut in pain, sometimes in bits of brilliant color, sometimes in muted tones. I put aside the old patterns but provide new improvisations from them.

Each piece of fabric in our creation is a remnant of life experience. One woman had eight children; another's husband had cancer. My David once lived here. I continue to feel his presence. I still see him seated at his grandfather's desk with the carved moldings. To cut and shape the right word in our caring and personal communications is like making a crazy quilt; only a certain irregularity of color will enhance the whole. Joined together into a quilt of extraordinary value, we are bordered by more than fat quarters and half square triangles.

Our quilts are often unfinished, and the academic observation that the mythic journey of life is, for women, more like a series of different walks definitely applies to me. Our stories are always sacred, filling up the blank pages of singular, tuckered-out lives.

For me, sometimes the sight of a light blue Dodge pickup plucks me back to ordinary frontseat memories, or the shredded wheat on the grocery shelf calls out to be brought home for David's breakfast. But I still forge on with a mysterious uplift of genuine thankfulness to include, as the Canterbury minister recently stated in his newsletter: "for all those who helped to make us who we are."

The Universe Gifts Me with Courage in All Things
I cherish my own courage. I salute myself for the brave action
I undertake in my life. I focus with clarity and appreciation on
the
choices I have made which have required courage and determination. I
applaud myself for my strength and my daring
        —*Julia Cameron*

VIII. Identity

Going to a writer's workshop on gorgeous Star Island in the summer of 2011 had been a clear sign of the birthing of a courageous new me. Years after David's death, this experience, much broader than I expected, seemed to provide incentive that spurred on so much self-discovery. It was risky in many ways to someone my age, because of the high level of physical exertion needed to get around a rocky island. But the days had been packed with all sorts of new challenges and exercises. Surrounded by soaring gulls, salty breezes, and quaint little anchored boats nodding in the peaceful harbor, we students enthusiastically responded to sensitive teaching techniques. We prepared to return to the mainland with its now siren call to hammer out the changing messages of our hearts and hands.

The identity issue that has haunted me through my lifetime has shrunk in importance. Although adolescence was once supposed to be the key age to have identity problems, I believe that extended life spans now demand that we reevaluate meanings as we live out a diversity of issues, including observations from within. Of course a little self-knowledge can go a long way!

As my days without David stretch on, I decide that the years with David as wife and lover had created awareness of my first authentic identity. In the era before David, I had believed that achievement was prime, and that behaving myself meant always living in vague fears or retaliations. Only later did I learn that life is not an automatic reward system. What had been held up to me as perfect (I still hate that word) didn't exist. It's okay to sometimes reflect, to skip the conventional, and to do things out of season. As an immature youth I had craved attention and focused on how I felt about my physical appearance. Too tall? Too thin? Feet too big? I hadn't yet learned that the limelight of life could be harrowing as well as glamorous when issues of intangible things like privacy, justice, freedom, and loving commitment had not taken precedence over current fad or style or cultural norm. Having felt like just an observer frozen by rules, feeling mute and incomplete, I became mesmerized by this man who didn't care about petty things, seldom judged others, and pursued friendships that were not based on what he was wearing. For him it was authenticity that came through even if his clothing was disheveled, wrinkled, or just plain hilarious. After what felt like a lifetime of strict do's and don'ts, oughts and musts, his presence beside me in the moment gave me the courage to let go and shut down the influence of certain old controlling patterns of authority in my childhood and early adulthood.

Yes, rules are there, but they have changed. To be a nice person or to be liked by everyone is no longer a primary goal. Behavioral admonitions have been replaced by current realistic need, as in "get to the dump before it closes at three," or, "why not check on the friend with that new medical diagnosis before her nap time?"

Then there had been the joy and relief of finding someone who understood me and seemed to see in me something appealing and simmering! His presence, his calm, his steady manner—even his positive responses to a terminal condition—had shown me another way of living life. Thank God. I stop and assess the delinquent "now."

I could actually start my new identity search by resorting to a touch of lighthearted satire. I know that, like most folks, I am simply the doughnut hole in the medical system, a carry-all bag, a "zipcode," the slow riser, a person who by watching the Andy of Mayberry reruns slips back for a few minutes into an era when things felt safe, innocent, and peaceful. And while a tattoo is now considered a reliable form of identity, I don't have one. Inside I am still the girl who swirled her ballerina skirt to dance to Vaughn Monroe at the Melrose

YMCA, swam that first stroke at Girl Scout camp on Damariscotta Lake, and will always be haunted by the sound of wild geese veering south.

But I continue this late life quest by researching what experts say about self-esteem. Where had my lack of it come from? I knew that while my parents loved me, I developed neither confidence in myself nor awareness of my own personal needs. I especially remember my childhood speculation about marriage and mothers, and that a house-wife seemed to mean ugly, loose dresses with slip straps showing while looking up at the kitchen wall clock to see if it was time to peel the potatoes and get the "supper going." A nurturing kind of love was absent, and I remained silent, with others' welfare always primary. Locked in rigid expectations, the idea of forgiveness was absent, and words of praise scarce, compliments a surprise. But unknowingly I learned about healthy cultural attitudes toward seniors, which led me to graduate work and creating workshops on aging. Sometimes, now when I have the passing impression that a neighbor speaks to me as if I were a real and capable person, I conclude that I might at last be making progress in the awareness of any singular value. But in Connecticut and New Hampshire, unfinished basements were the only places for sewing paraphernalia.

Now as I gain confidence and learn to speak out, I like to speculate about what had been other women's abilities to adapt. For example, when women went west in wagons in the nineteenth century and had only one change of underwear, Grandma's quilt, and a chicken or two, were they mulling over the right way to say, "I need a bath"?

My study of self-esteem then led me to thinking about whether there had ever been a role model while I was growing up. Yes, there was clearly a Mrs. Lewis, a pastor's wife who, though denied a semi-nary education because of her gender, was smart and accepting and smiling, with a magical ability to reach out to our teen age Sunday school class that included a gawky girl like me!

Actually if I look in the mirror now, I frighten myself. What happened? Did I waste time? At age eighty I now know that any identity is definitely tied to my age. Good character and flexibility, not appearance, are important. Living alone has never been a problem, but now it is becoming an issue; the body sometimes says "no." I have even dared to research some assisted living facilities.

The concerns about myself are growing, not because I became more selfish but because when the aging body slows down or quits, many levels of change come into our lives. Relationship changes are the hardest. Friends disappear, relatives die, neighbors come and go. But there are other random identity changes. Here are a few:

I don't drive at night.

I resigned from the condo board.

Shopping for food means pre-mixed, picked up, or ready to pop in the oven.

I try to truly listen to my peers when they chatter and veer off into this and that because I too live alone, often with no place to vent.

I seldom turn on the TV before 6 pm.

With relief, I no longer lift and carry wood for the fireplace because I got smart and put in a gas unit for emergencies.

I divide my precious days into rigid time compartments, giving me a sense of security and priority. Creative writing is best done in the morning. Then mindless stitching on a quilt is best done between three and five in the afternoon.

I go to church on Sunday one hour before services begin in order to find an adjacent parking space, and then sit in the car and read for a while. Gone are the days when early to rise meant looking for a child's missing shoe before dashing for the car. (We once headed for home, leaving a four-year-old daughter Laurie standing on the church corner.)

I am on the alert for small things that become big fixations.

I am working on developing patience because I have learned that the stubborn New England tendency of using the hasty trial and error method of learning may not be the best way to approach problems.

My faith practice, attuned to the metronome of loss, deliberately lifts up silence as part of my every day. I listen and weed and wrestle with God.

The biggest challenge of my age and so-called identity is how to communicate to my children that I am no longer the parent of their childhood, and will in turn require advice and care from others. (I had always felt sorry for people who had to do something for me!) At the same time, I look at my grown children, the five grandchildren, and the four great-grandchildren, and am overwhelmed with thankfulness. My three are grown-up, sensitive, reliable members of society. I just get irritated at times when some young adult tells me I remind them of their grandmother who shingled the roof yesterday! Am I not more than physical expertise? In between my sensible shoes and my gray matter, there is some wisdom learned from life experience. How do I best use it?

Thank God some of us aging folks are refusing the stereotypical definition of "old."

Consider the elder who took her grandson on an Elderhostel trip, that vibrant church lady who went off to help the folks in Zimbabwe, the hospice volunteer who cheers up the elderly shut-in, and of course the masses of us with knitting neuroses and quilting mania providing handmade and colorful necessities for daily living. Compassion carried out in one way or another.

In the remainder of my senior identity search I guess I will always be rebelling at something, as in not wanting to sing "Jingle Bell Rock" in the middle of October, or questioning the working hours of my grandchildren, that make it difficult to get together for visits. But I also recall with surprise that first time when my then husband canceled out of my birthday plans because of church business, and I had the courage to declare I would go by myself, and did. That incident in turn reminded me of the time when I defied strict rules from the town fathers after a blizzard, and with a friend jumped into my blue Volkswagon bug and took groceries to our stranded mothers, who lived in a neighboring town.

Maybe there's hope for me yet! Maybe I was not as passive as I originally thought. Maybe over the years I've been too critical of myself. So I become more accepting of myself, and at times take my own turn at saying "good grief!" Just yesterday it dawned on me that I was the one who found the rental camp on the lake; I was the one who discovered a place (Cape Porpoise, Maine) to celebrate finishing my master's degree; I was the one who searched out another spot to replace our summer beach house. Except I will probably always be frugal. (Wasn't David lucky to have such a frugal woman for a wife!) When I now look at the increase in the price of calico stamped on the end of the bolt, the decision is made for me. I will "make do" with the boxes of scraps in the basement.

I like to believe that the calendar has become less a prop, but of course it's necessary for all those doctor's appointments.

I am careful to not judge myself as to what I did or did not do. I remind myself of the value of just being, that I did the best I could at the time.

I am aware that certain comments were never digested or applied, as, for example, David's "you work harder than any person I've ever known!" Flattering, of course, but later finding myself evaluating any truth there, in realizing that those in the arts can have a level of concentration that is overdone. (My pleasure in the arts had nothing to do with money, praise or acclaim. It's the inner satisfaction that could bring pleasure to others, but is primarily a form of self-expression or challenge.) I am now keenly aware, as poet Denise Levertov states, that there is interaction between the journey of art and the journey of faith; every work of art is an adventure into the unknown that supplies a unique kind of solace. Even writing, according to author Edna O'Brien when a guest of radio host Diane Rheim, is a confronting of the self. I could never have completed a final essay exam in graduate school if I hadn't, at the same time, been working on a certain quilt for my Star Island friend Ginny.

Any new identity must include what gives me pleasure, as in an occasional TV special such as *My Life as a Turkey*, a story of possibility, of human closeness to nature. Or time for afternoon tea with my neighbor Arlene or lunch with a new friend Dot. Or the holding of contented baby Owen at a jolly family birthday party. Or the finding of a forgotten piece of memorabilia from David's life. The great thing about photos is that people in them never go totally away. Seeing them when leafing through a scrapbook means they are still around, not really gone.

Most of all, I am a person who has discovered that she cannot live without music. Yes, piano practice that my folks had provided taught me a level of discipline that gave me the guts to hang in there when things got tough. But it's the listening to certain kinds of music that fills the vacant moments, invites me into their tempo, brings back associations, and most of all exhibits order and beauty. The purity of tone can refocus me from the rocky ground of pain and loss to the good and joyful and soothing. But I also buy a Gilbert and Sullivan CD to occasionally bring back the carefree mood of the British musical comedy team that had brought David and me so much pleasure.

Who I am is now less important than how I lived my life. I'm not papier-mâché or weighty granite; not quilted, carved, or hand-blown. I'm flesh and blood, still capable of choosing whom or what I can serve, and I acknowledge more openly the centrality of faith in my life. And I enjoy a momentary giggle as I remember how David had described his religious life as "spotty" on his "advanced care planning guide." The long caregiving experience tamed me and taught me and allowed me precious time with a man I truly loved.

As I get ready for a yard sale, I am suddenly reminded of a similar experience many years ago when my first husband and I had an auction of all our belongings "except for the books and our children" we would later cheerily chirp, so that he could return to school to get another graduate degree. Yes, material things had been sparse, but we were rather happy at the mere thought of returning to New England and what would be a new chapter in our lives. Now, in the so-called fifth season of my life, I can also again let go of some things without strong regrets. For some crazy reason it's fun to picture that chair or teapot in someone else's living room. Moreover, if I keep it,

I'll have to dust it. My life is boiling down more and more to the simple and basic, and that's okay with me.

I hear a new voice, as poet Mary Oliver says. My own. Yes, I find I'm glad about many things, especially glad that I was able to keep David at home with me during those last years.

I decide that as an adult I have had two major roles, not identities: a clergy wife and a wifely caregiver, sometimes feeling like nothing but a renegade witness to the pains and passions of living. Now what matters? Matters? Matters? Yes, Gilbert and Sullivan, you always keep up with truths! While any talk of a legacy statement smacks of the risky return to "oughts and musts," I pray that the acceptance and valuing of the self will matter and will lead to a broader understanding and specific ways of caring for others. I am still on the gradual move, alone or with community, at least "to see more clearly" as the thirteenth chapter of First Corinthians suggests.

IX. Waking

It is nine years since David left me, but God has not forgotten me, the woman who gnashed and bitched over her losses as she pondered concern for family and church. Now with time to closely examine the past, a new awareness of losses, blessings, lessons learned, and experiences digested reveal surprises as to where meaning was found.

After my rather strict upbringing and the sickness and death of two husbands, my story as a single woman continues, David's love of life forever instrumental in my life changes.

I did try reviewing the kinds of losses that change our ways of living. Of course the world wants us to pretend, wisecrack, ignore, and even smile while bearing the pain or learning to juggle new kinds of love. But I needed to move from regimented behavior, as in two hours of piano practice per day, and regular night meetings or church activities, to believing that sometimes wisdom and creativity and service to others—family, neighbor, or far away stranger—may come first.

My sister Mary Ella's deteriorating physical condition had meant selling her family home. I had watched my grown nieces Cindy and Pam struggle with the multiple decisions concerning my sister's condition: helpful home care, VA nursing, neighbors' gifts, doctor appointments, and then research into assisted living with its paper-work evaluations, meal quality, financial comparison, and the placing of pets. With my sister's death came another numbing loss, unleashing those same familiar feelings of helplessness and grief.

All of this grieving uncovered the reality of my own denial about options. Yes, my turn is coming, but the memory of the dismantling of the big house is still brewing. The "where," the "near what," and the "with who" is daunting. Just losing a place for get togethers can be a loss of surprising depth for the majority of Americans who now live in reduced space. For me, because of my tiny condo, Christmas dinner last year meant a trip to the Portsmouth Sheraton, where Santa greeted the crowd of us, high chairs were provided, and the children and grandchildren, as summertime Star Island voyagers, could look out at the big familiar vista of the Thomas Laighton ferry docked for the winter. Or consider another example of loss. After the death of my first husband, and at the recommendation of staff at Massachusetts General Hospital, I had become a subject of the award-winning TV program on loss, *Begin With Good-bye,* hosted by Eli Wallach. I had represented the widow, while others shared different experiences such as job loss, and the loss of a body part. If I were the author of that script now, I would include the loss of a beloved pet because when Amos, my cat, died seven years after David I again felt stabbed by pain. Watching the cat take his last breath at the veterinary clinic, with its displays of medical products, friendly staff, and anxious clients on leashes, I knew that, as with David's absence, there would be no more warm welcomes on future arrivals home.

When Carolyn and I packed for the annual Labor Day escape to the camp in the lakes region last year, we had to brace for the fact that it would be our last time there. Another kind of loss. The owner had been forced to sell. So my daughter made our last stay at the lake bearable. She hauled the drinking water, prepared dinners, made my bed. She swam laps and sang now and then in joyful exuberance as the sky did its spectacular peach thing at dusk. I sat on the tiny private beach hoping to permanently absorb the sights and sound of the waterfront vista where I had been annually calmed, supported, and energized, and where the evening meant sewing with lovely fabrics purchased at our favorite store, *Keepsake Quilting,* in nearby Center Harbor. My help clearly came from a loving daughter not just "from the hills" as per the famous biblical quote.

But as I note the numerous other but more subtle losses—time, independence, and others too numerous to mention here—the paper-work continues to pile up. While I'm aware I'd rather brood over the choice of a dazzling background for that Project Linus quilt, I pay a few bills and scribble a reminder as to exactly what I have learned, for example, about redefining a productive day away from an economic and status base to the inner working and needs of heart and soul.

I have learned that there is a sanctity of place that is never lost. The beach house, the lakefront cottage, and the Star Island Confer-ence Center provided three powerful backdrops for our marriage and all the meaningful interplay of people's lives. Yes, you could say they are landscapes of sadness now. But they are also lighthearted action snapshots in my mind: Bill hitting a homer again at Star's Thursday baseball game; Laurie gracing an afternoon tea party for the young children at the beach house; Carolyn swimming circles around the float at the lakefront cottage. The seagulls, the rocking chairs, the reflective time, and the diverse range of interesting people are still available. Then one day I find a way to negotiate my section of famous Route 4. For those who frequent the winding miles from Portsmouth to Concord and back, this can be a memory lane of surprising plea-sure. Consider:

See that dip in the road? My friend Harriet's Christmas tree lights up her dock every year, bringing joy to passers-by on a snowy evening.

Going east down the road is the famous Wagon Hill Farm where David and I had watched Cecil the dog joyfully cavort and run free. Or heading west toward Lee there is the sprawling estate that once included browsing llamas as well as lilacs.

There's the campus of Coe-Brown, which demands that I slow down.

What was once a restaurant now invites dental care.

There's the white clapboard Higher Ground Baptist Church.

Our favorite covered vegetable stand.

Johnson's Ice Cream Bar.

Northwood's tornado damage of 2012.

The amazing *Piece Time Puzzles* store, housed in a barn where we also find gifts.

The Route 202 turnoff to my sister's Waterboro camp.

The memorable place on the hill where one late summer evening, returning to Canterbury from the beach house, David and I had pulled over to view a spectacular display of northern lights.

The antiques shop where I had bought an enchanting tilt top table.

The Epsom Circle, where a policeman is proudly remembered.

The rest stop now closed.

The pink house that calls out to sample its wares.

The turn-off to Route 106 and the Makris Fish Restaurant, where my sister and I had often met for a delicious lunch.

Finally, on approaching Concord, the distant sight off to the right of the Swenson Granite complex, representing such a marvelous piece of New Hampshire history.

I am so thankful for these ordinary places, which are not totally gone, although some of the names have changed slightly. They are still there for me—the laughter, the friendly greetings, and the wonderful fresh air. Places not of luxury but of a variety of moods and circumstances—peaceful, hectic, historic, or nostalgic.

The intensity of pain and loss followed by looking back has led me to believe that David was a composite of positive attributes previously missing from my entire adult life. How could I have been so lucky as to meet and know him? Because the steady and calm approach to life was what I needed, my life with David bordered on the miraculous.

I have also discovered that I truly love the state in which I live. It is so easy to paint New Hampshire in folksy, nostalgic terms when in reality we are an up-to-date colorful landscape, within easy proximity to Boston area perks and a modest seacoast that is often ignored. Less congested than most states, New Hampshire provides the possibility of working at home while viewing majestic mountain ranges.

Thank goodness that storyteller Fritz Wetherbee keeps coming with his delightful historic thumbnail-sized vignettes each night on the TV *NH Chronicle* series. The editors of the giant one-volume *Encyclopedia of New England* claim that New Hampshire has no distinct identity, in contrast to Maine with its lobsters and Massachusetts with its beans. (Well, right now we have the distinction of all-female political representation.)

The future of my beloved state may surprise even us. Tourists will of course find changes in our scenic vista. There are NASCAR races and rock-climbing camps to add to the once pristine lakes, ski slopes, town meetings, mills, and campgrounds. The Oceanic Hotel on glorious Star Island is now more open to the public.

What I have learned includes the fact that questions will always be around, but they tend to be of increased depth of meaning as I age and as I experience a global awareness of things like starvation, terrorist attacks, climate change, and homelessness. (Kind of a big change from childhood questions like, "why does Daddy have his own chair?") I continue to question the concept of closure for those grieving, question the language of today, question how grandchildren will afford a good education, question how to lessen the aloneness of another. I dare to ask if I supplied good support for David, or expressed my kind of love for him often enough. I dare to ask if memories are always trustworthy. I ask philosophical questions like "what is a balanced life?" or squirm over hidden questions like "can a society that values self-reliance, personal freedom, and careerism reconcile itself to the realities of dependence, diminished autonomy and responsibility for others?" (As stated by the authors of *Taking Care.*) Or why didn't I more easily accept the changed daily lifestyle that his illness imposed upon us? We still had each other then, to have and to hold. Now dawns the realization that what had been the underlying emotional question as I had scribbled those retorts and exclamations was "who really cares about me?"

In my search for truth, I read how religious historian Karen Armstrong acknowledged the negative effect of rigidity in her early church life when she was a nun, yet spiraled herself to a better understanding of living. This encourages me. The institutional church was the place where I met the love of my life, the man with all those endearing traits that fulfilled the deepest longing of my lonely heart. What went before in my disjointed spiritual journey nourishes me. Less in the way of doctrine, more in the struggle through pain and loss as I learn to see God in certain others.

So as I rethink the institutional church, tea and cookies and a two-minute devotional for small groups probably won't be enough. Sitting in a small circle of secular women without warning I sometimes have an urge to reach out, hold the hands of those on my left and right, and pray. Good grief! Another of those deep-seated questions: Does life become one long prayer? As a writer it is easy to note various traits, as there will always be those who want to sing only the old tunes, and there will always be tearful breakdowns over the increases in church building maintenance costs. There will always be church suppers. I remember the rush to get home with some leftovers. I had left my large red purse on the roof of the car, only to be tailed for miles by a police car. There was a phone call at home later to say they had found my purse smelling like cheese! The church will always be going through its own kind of timely struggle to stay alive, minister to, and identify itself. As events flash on the TV screen in endless depiction of fears and misery both worldwide and in our own *Mr. Rogers Neighborhood,* I become aware that more could be done to relieve the sick and the wounded of any faith. As our dedicated adult choir witnesses to the congregation every Sunday, I find reasons for hope. I acknowledge that the institutional church is a place where caring can be carried out in a million different ways. The church is a giant network of persons able but maybe needing "how to be helpful" to be spelled out. They are capable of becoming caregivers to the world, but they crave authentic leadership and need to choose some form of meaningful communal rituals as priorities change.

My first husband was a fine man who gave generously to all parishioners. He was not tuned in to innovative programming or business management, but he set his own impossible goals, such as his wish for personal visitation in all church homes a minimum of twice a year. Seeing people was his primary concern. His own sickness and death opened up his ability to lead powerful seminars on death and dying.

In spite of years in the ministry with my first husband, it was David, who by his quiet, humble ways, taught me how life is meant to be lived. He didn't try to save the world. Just by his noncritical attitude, his steady example and forthright directness, he made simple kindness and acceptance prime. I find it especially interesting that reflection brings the realization that the death of my first husband was followed by travel into wide-open places, as in a windjammer cruise out of Camden, Maine. And the death of my second husband brought a terrifying sense of aloneness that eventually led to a wider understanding of the so-called human condition. Perhaps I could express it best by saying that it was husband Bill's call to ministry and David's humble but gregarious self that led me to the simple aware-ness that it is people who touch our lives and make the difference. (Sometimes now I think it's friends who keep me going, although last week one friend died, one was diagnosed with Alzheimer's, and one moved away.) True love followed by self-knowledge brings new awareness of others.

So now I do not begin the day by reading the obituaries, the "who died and who didn't." I want to know more about living things. Grandson Ian just bought a quaint old house, Jayne had throat surgery in Boston, Leah is putting herself through college and has just accepted a diamond from Adam, baby Owen was baptized on Star Island, Lyla started first grade. Carolyn takes on treasurer work for a UCC Star Conference, Laurie cares for her four grandchildren on Monday, Friday, and Saturday. (Her childhood wish to be Mrs. Walton has almost come true!) And I continue to marvel at others' stories of happiness and joy, as well as those of resilience and sacrifice, and difficult facts that depict a large diversity of need and condition and caregiving circumstances, parent/child relationships, disability, dementia, and PTSD. In our own extended families, we are now mourning the death of niece Whitney's baby and granddaughter Kayley's husband Eric.

All kinds of people have been part of my life, each with powerful resources. There was the elderly woman who sat by my bed day after day in the hospital when my baby died back in Iowa. An amazing unconventional woman who reached out to an ignorant young minister's wife from cold New England with her gift of a sticky recipe card for Winifred's White Frosting, which brings the Kentucky hillside alive to me. Friend Brenda whose family gave up all Thanksgivings to pack and deliver the Stamford Meals on Wheels dinners. The last gentle Shaker sisters, with their modest greeting of peace and tranquility to each and every museum guest. My sister Mary Ella, who, after the death of my first husband, drove every Thursday from Concord, New Hampshire, to Lynnfield, Massachusetts, to visit with me. Perhaps if we all realized how much one person can influence one other, we would devote less time to hasty messaging and more to responding in gentle, personal ways.

David and I were blessed with a loving family and friends: my immediate family—Laurie and Rick, Carolyn and Bill, Ian, Steve, Christina, Ryan, Kayley, Lyla, Jacob, Leah, Jayne, and now baby Owen; some New Hampshire Swensons—Malcolm and Barbara and Davy, Andy and Mary, Kurt and Kevin's families; Betty and all the nieces and nephews and cousins too numerous to mention out west and in Washington, DC. Quality relationships sustain, but impersonal acquaintances maintained via cyberspace alone may not.

I admit that in the tiredness and endless routines and worries about lack of future time for personal dreams, I had forgotten that demands and restructure wouldn't be forever. I remind myself that at Christmas we all sing "acquainted with grief." It is easy to get discouraged when I live alone, when I miss David's "good morning, sweetheart" or when a new medical condition rears its unwelcome head.

I go back to Melrose with my son to visit my friend and former neighbor Laura Crouss, now age ninety-five. She has just moved into a senior housing facility that she, as a young church board member, had been instrumental in talking the town into building. If we all do our small part, change is made.

This year my son sends an Easter card with the verse "God is alive in everything" and I am able to silently say, yes, yes! My mantra today becomes "glimpses of truth thou hast for me" or perhaps "I go to prepare place for you." From fear and frustrations to faith and freedom and possibility.

I might not be the best little tree, Dad, but I believe that the artist in each of us will reveal that people are united by various ways of expressing their love. To live a balanced life of outreach and reflection is both an art and a goal. For me, now I hear a different drummer. Even at my age, I must continue to listen, search, and question if I am to grow!

X. Living Again

L ife fills up again.

Precious reflections of my children are especially sweet: Billy reciting the presidents, backward; Carolyn learning to play the cello; Laurie doing cartwheels across the lawn.

Humorous epitaphs on gravestones provide laughter again: "going but know not where," "walked with God till transplanted."

Keeping my own body repaired or at least upright is a full-time task, but I approach it with a different attitude. I can snicker at the e-mail list entitled "Somersworth Medical Directory" that arrived yesterday: DILATE, to live alone; BOWEL, a deep dish; ARTERY, the study of fine paintings; POST OPERATIVE, a letter carrier.

My own recent medical agenda expands. While my actual medical care is excellent, an unpredictable series of where and when is in order. Last week I had my yearly physical as well as a regular checkup with my cardiologist. (He's settled in his brand-new office after we patients chased him between temporary locations, here to there.) That was the same week of my annual eye exam. Last Tuesday I drove to Concord to see my dermatologist, having spent a significant period of my life in the sun (I noted that the familiar pink house on Route 4 is now purple!) On Wednesday I got up early to drive to my health center in Portsmouth for the blood test I was supposed to have had for that physical. In the afternoon of the same day I got a call from the hospital in Dover about scheduling some test, and learn that the hospital now owns a new facility, which I am told might be convenient in the future. The following day I made an appointment to meet with a specialist to address my spinal stenosis and pain in my right leg. (The epiderals last year had been helpful, but after the exposé about them, I am leery.) My front tooth dropped into my Cheerios yesterday. You could say that the trauma I experience from immersion in the medical world has receded some, although my age group always guarantees surprises.

In spare time between appointments (after ordering new eyeglasses from what seems like a thousand choices and at an unbelievable cost), and after thanking God my teeth are not in line for a checkup right now, and, aside from appointments for the car and the cat, my neighbor Arlene and I find time to compare medical notes on the phone. We end up laughing as our tales of woe seem to be part of all days.

Arlene is presently using David's walker as she recoups from a fall, and her husband has been diagnosed with pneumonia, but they are determined to attend their sixty-fifth Dartmouth class reunion and do! I tell her about my recent sighting out back of my condo of a Great Blue Heron and a young kitten having a strange conversation at the water's edge. No one got hurt, but it was fun to imagine what the linguistic exchange could be like. Then we switch to the topic of books. I still find time to hunker down with Sonia Sotomayor's heartening autobiography, which uplifts me with her courage and stamina. And I share how I found time to view the scintillating TV series about presidents' wives and their wide variety of abilities to adapt, revealing strength on so many levels.

I still make quilts for my grandchildren, still gobble up peanut butter and tomato sandwiches, still read the King James version of the Christmas story, still love Mary Poppins' free spirit, and still remember how Amos the cat could fill the empty spaces in my life with his own kind of loving. So I make regular visits to the local SPCA until I find a gorgeous female named Gnosis who promises to be an affectionate lap cat. When I jovially taunt God to give me a sign as to whether this is the feline companion for me, I find the dictionary definition of her name—"knowledge of spiritual things"—to be just the ticket, and proceed to rename her Mildred. She now settles down to watch her own TV favorites, like the "Too Cute" series on *Animal Planet*.

You can see I am returning to mundane everyday things, like stockpiling flashlight batteries, practicing frugality, humming snatches of hymn tunes that never die, viewing the gentle deer moving silently across the lawn, and making some new rules of my own, like keeping three things for my essential living in every room: a flashlight, a pair of scissors, and an extra pair of glasses. I also take time to remember the joyful get-togethers playing bridge with friend Diane as she dealt with her ALS condition cheerfully.

Maybe I'm recovering my normality as I haul my own batch of necessities in the back of my trusty Subaru. My second home? I add library books next to three beach hats, extra sneakers, a chocolate stash, an emergency blanket, and a windbreaker. Sometimes I get an oil change. Sometimes I wash the exterior, remembering fondly the dog Cecil's grim expression when water gushed overhead in the car wash. And every month I make another car payment and remember David beside me in the Peugeot on our various outings.

I don't like the idea of becoming the matriarch, however. I don't like a world without my sister Mary Ella. I don't want to outlive everyone. I already feel like a mere storage unit since niece Ellen passed on the last boxes of Clark family albums from my brother's barn. But I am so thankful for the grown grandchildren and their little ones Lyla, Jacob, Ryan, and Owen, who are bringing their own rays of light into my aging years.

As we live longer and care is accessible, medical agendas will demand a major part of our living. A surprising portion of our lives will be spent in sporadic discussion and intense involvement with the needs of others, many of whom live alone. I know that the strain on family life caused by giving constant physical and emotional care can make balanced care a precarious business. The "how long" is kept hidden as months stretch to years as we caregivers secretly wonder when she or he will wear out.

Health care is not as glamorous as TV may lead us to believe. It is a way of life for thousands of dedicated employees, doctors, nurses, aides and volunteers who seem happily capable of drifting about and through while the rest of us may cringe, tiptoe, obey, fear, follow, and sometimes get better. Only now do I realize that much of my anger at the medical system was a coverup for my anger at losing the man who had become the center of my life.

I believe that the word caregiver will continue to point to our confusion and to incorrect interpretation. With more than 34 million unpaid caregivers providing care to someone age eighteen or older who is ill or has a disability (according to AARP), maybe if it is defined as a privilege, we would see people flocking to provide helpful behavior. (This makes me think of my childhood habit of rowing my brother around the lake so he could fly cast for trout. As I tended to worship anything he put his mind to, I only later concluded that he had made the chore sound like a privilege.) Though health care is often viewed as only a financial problem, we may be the ones who must bring the issue into the spotlight, create better routines, try to pay more attention to new medical information, and speak out concerning opportunities for quality care. Few home caregivers are aware of community support systems and the need for trained, fairly paid home care workers. Already we are seeing young adults caught up in carrying dual roles of caregiving, as in the dilemma of caring for both newborns and dying parents at the same time. While we can never be prepared for this role, it may surprisingly bring talents/ abilities to light.

While the future requires support from both genders I want to say to the reader not to buy the subtle cultural message that as a woman you must do it all. Trying to do everything leaves little time and energy for personal time. The effects of stress on such women is only now being studied, the effect of giving long-term care now being fully tabulated. To take your own pulse during the caregiving process is not easy. Faced with multiple tasks both physically and emotionally draining, the ability to stop and evaluate is not as auto-matic as later advice might be. How we treat ourselves as female care-givers is primary. Illness in my childhood had meant fear and false expectations, while for others there are countless memories of coura-geous role models. (A relative just recently said that I should have had more help. Well, it was my fault. I should have asked for it.) If you turn to certain web sites now, you can find lists of tips on caring for yourself. This includes things like watching for signs of depression and rewarding yourself. Respite organizations now exist to give family caregivers a needed break.

I realize there are many other issues of caregiving that my ramblings have omitted or are ignored or denied, as noted in increasing numbers of magazine and newspaper articles on financial scams, fear of abandonment, dealing with difficult family members, physical abuse, and failing mental capacity. The world needs sensitive persons, paid or unpaid, churchy or secular. If you need help with the whole idea of compassion, read Karen Armstrong's *Twelve Steps to a Compassionate Life.*

We must not write people off because they are labeled sick or disabled. We must give others a chance to still grow and model for us about living and dying. If we strike them down in faceless categories at the first sign of an inconvenience, disfigurement, or diagnosis, we are failing them as well as ourselves. Just consider the military folk returning with all sorts of injuries that need attention, and love.

Aside from a doctor's office, a conference room, or a lonely hospital corner, we must provide places where care comes from the heart. Just knowing people's stories of joy and loss can kindle under-standing and empathy and some forms of action.

Some people like to point out to me that I've "had" two loving husbands, meaning, don't complain. They're right. I've been fortunate, and I've finally accepted the fact that life never gets tidied up like a tree farm—predictable, straight. I admit that in the tiredness and endless routines, I had forgotten that emptiness and absence wouldn't be forever. Maybe I had an antiquated view of illness. The world of sickness was a world I knew little about. It was difficult for me to accept help, but with increased involvement in the present medical world has come more knowledge for the future.

Sometimes I don't think I can start over again: make a home out of a void, find new doctors and services, visit a different church. But sometimes I even reflect on all those parsonages, recalling their unique characteristics rather than their problematic issues. Other times, even restricted living has an attraction if I can keep an open mind.

I also sometimes wonder what in life stays the same. Today what's familiar is the regularity of death because on September eighth it is David's brother Andy, the Swenson patriarch, who leaves us, who had brought us together with his wonderful birthday parties and generous nature.

While I live in a housing complex where the howl of arriving ambulances is somewhat regular, I continue to evaluate my own gifts and how they fit amidst others in spite of my slowing down. Now with my new attitude about life, I can admit that I had always projected never being needy myself, and being five foot ten often fooled the world with a "you can't hurt me."

If I had a single top-notch close up photo of David to treasure with him it would be of a quiet evening sitting together in the cozy end of our giant dining room, browsing through his Union Leader, and me sewing on a current project, or him bursting into the kitchen with a bouquet in one hand, a small bag of groceries in the other, and a blush of pure joy on his face. He loved to bring me flowers, and often did. Whether they came from a fancy florist or a grocery store vendor, buying them for me brought him as much pleasure as it did me. My day of boring sameness or kitchen drudgery was put on hold as I greeted him with smiles and kisses. His whim of posies changed us both. Or maybe I'd choose the photo of David happily taking off for discount Tuesday, toting his ancient skis that qualified for exhibition at the New Hampshire Ski Museum, complete with faded Goldwater stickers stuck on top!

Now at age eighty, I find a new-for-me metaphor of life. The word "stone," and its connotation with durability and strength, sounds comparable to character and the ability to guide. What I had not understood about the Great Stone Face as a child had been made clear. It meant another musical mantra, as in "like your rocks of towering grandeur, make me strong and sure." So as I sit in the car overlooking Wallis Sands Beach, the sound of water washing its regular beat against our rugged shoreline seems enough to heal my aging and lonely spirit.

Reflecting once again, I recall the trip with David to the Mount Rushmore memorial when he was sent there on a consulting job. We viewed the massive presidential faces—a sixty-foot-high rendition of George Washington, Thomas Jefferson, Teddy Roosevelt, and Abraham Lincoln carved into granite there in the Black Hills of South Dakota. It attracts nearly three million tourists a year.

From the lone lookout of the New Hampshire Great Stone Face to the illusion of crowded beachfront houses as faces at Wells, Maine, to this giant quartet of presidential facades in South Dakota, it is the form of the human face that represents the deepest of communication to the millions looking up for inspiration to carry on. Friends, relatives, parishioners, strangers. We learn about God through the lives of others, don't we?

Love as lasting, chiseled stone promises the presence of others to impact our ordinary lives, like what had come to David and I—a life-giving force, a union that can last forever. A move from loving to loss to grief to a gradual foggy return to everyday living exposes at last a surprising gratitude that mysteriously emerges as the universal theme that it is. Of course, the mature kind of love is not easy, preaches my UCC friend Reverend Jack Lynes. "To bless is to suffer," speaks the new Episcopal bishop of New Hampshire in a *Concord Monitor* interview.

The capacity to love never leaves us. It may falter as we hang in there, or hide its face when we are immersed in difficult times. But there is a divine spark, whatever our belief system, that resides out of sight, deep within. You can stomp on it, curse it, try to bury it, disclaim it, coat yourself with it, or carry it, forever making all that you do and say with it. With all those memories of family, relationships, and community, I find myself grateful.

David, David. My beloved. Thank you. Yes, the early death of my first husband left me with three teens and taxes, but your death left me with an everlasting perspective of a questing self and the knowledge that there is no right or wrong way to grieve.

And dear reader, with your own boundless gifts and stresses of daily living and dying, I hope that my humble story, from love to scribbled grief to the return of simple normality will help you to honestly face the caregivings and losses of tomorrow.

In final testimony, I just try to practice the presence of God, like Brother Lawrence, when doing the dishes, reminding myself that after being part of the waiting rooms of the world, and having been promised the gifts of the spirit, I am grounded at last, and while the cat's comforting little motorboat sounds provide background music, that is enough.

> I have noticed that even in the midst of the most profound spiritual darkness, there is ever in the centre of the soul a certain light of pure faith which is a most safe guide.
>
> —the Rev. Jean-Pierre de Caussade, *Abandonment to Divine Providence*